Epilepsy

AMERICAN ACADEMY OF NEUROLOGY (AAN)
Quality of Life Guides
Lisa M. Shulman, MD
Series Editor

Alzheimer's Disease
Paul Dash, MD, and Nicole Villemarette-Pittman, PhD

Amyotrophic Lateral Sclerosis
Robert G. Miller, MD, Deborah Gelinas, MD,
and Patricia O'Connor, RN

Epilepsy
Ilo E. Leppik, MD

Guillain-Barré Syndrome
Gareth John Parry, MD, and Joel S. Steinberg, MD

Migraine and Other Headaches
William B. Young, MD, and Stephen D. Silberstein, MD

Restless Legs Syndrome
Mark J. Buchfuhrer, MD, Wayne A. Hening, MD, PhD,
and Clete A. Kushida, MD, PhD

Peripheral Neuropathy
Norman Latov, MD, PhD

Stroke
Louis R. Caplan, MD

Understanding Pain
Harry J. Gould, III, MD, PhD

Epilepsy

A Guide to Balancing Your Life

ILO E. LEPPIK, MD

Professor,
College Pharmacy
Adjunct Professor
Department of Neurology
University of Minnesota Medical School
Minneapolis, Minnesota

LISA M. SHULMAN, MD

Series Editor

Associate Professor of Neurology
Rosalyn Newman Distinguished Scholar in Parkinson's Disease
Co-Director, Maryland Parkinson's Disease
and Movement Disorders Center
University of Maryland School of Medicine
Baltimore, Maryland

Demos

New York

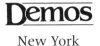

AAN PRESS
AMERICAN ACADEMY OF
NEUROLOGY

Library of Congress Cataloging-in-Publication Data

Leppik, Ilo E.
 Epilepsy / Ilo E. Leppik.
  p. cm. — (American Academy of Neurology (AAN) quality of life guides)
 Includes bibliographical references and index.
 ISBN-13: 978-1-932603-20-0 (pbk. : alk. paper)
 ISBN-10: 1-932603-20-4 (pbk. : alk. paper)
 1. Epilepsy—Popular works. I. Title.
 RC372.L462   2006
 616.8'53—dc22

                                                                2006021063

Special discounts on bulk quantities of Demos Medical Publishing books are available to corporations, professional associations, pharmaceutical companies, health care organizations, and other qualifying groups. For details, please contact:

Special Sales Department
Demos Medical Publishing
386 Park Avenue South, Suite 301
New York, NY 10016
Phone: 800-532-8663, 212-683-0072
Fax: 212-683-0118
Email: orderdept@demosmedpub.com

Printed in Canada

06 07 08 09 10   5 4 3 2 1

Contents

Contents

About the AAN Press
Quality of Life Guides

In the Spirit of the Doctor-Patient Partnership

THE BETTER-INFORMED PATIENT is often able to play a vital role in his or her own care. This is especially the case with neurologic disorders, for which effective management of disease can be promoted—indeed, *enhanced*—through patient education and involvement.

In the spirit of the partnership-in-care between physicians and patients, the American Academy of Neurology Press is pleased to produce a series of "Quality of Life" guides on an array of diseases and ailments that affect the brain and nervous system. The series, produced in partnership with Demos Medical Publishing, answers a number of basic and important questions faced by patients and their families.

Additionally, the authors, most of whom are physicians and all of whom are experts in the areas in which they write, provide a detailed discussion of the disorder, its causes, and the course it may follow. You also find strategies for coping with the disorder and handling a number of nonmedical issues.

The result: As a reader, you will be able to develop a framework for understanding the disease and become better prepared to manage the life changes associated with it.

About the American Academy of Neurology (AAN)

The American Academy of Neurology is the premier organization for neurologists worldwide. In addition to support of educational and scientific advances, the AAN—along with its sister organization, the AAN Foundation—is a strong advocate of public education and a leading supporter of research for breakthroughs in neurologic patient care.

More information on the activities of the AAN is available on our website, www.aan.com. For a better understanding of common disorders of the brain, as well as to learn about people living with these disorders, please turn to the AAN Foundation's website, www.thebrainmatters.org.

ABOUT NEUROLOGY AND NEUROLOGISTS

Neurology is the medical specialty associated with disorders of the brain and central nervous system. Neurologists are medical doctors with specialized training in the diagnosis, treatment, and management of patients suffering from neurologic disease.

Lisa M. Shulman, MD
Series Editor,
AAN Press Quality of Life Guides

Foreword

EPILEPSY IS ONE OF THE MOST common neurological disorders, and one poorly understood by both medical and nonmedical people since earliest recorded history. This is unfortunate because the outcome of treatment is often dependent on participation by the patient and family even more than other chronic neurologic disorders. The importance of active patient knowledge and participation in care is not unlike type 1 insulin-dependent diabetes mellitus.

Educational materials often include texts with much more detail or science than can be readily understood by patients and their families, or consist of superficial pamphlets and cartoons that significantly underestimate the interest and intelligence of the patients. The Internet offers educational opportunities, but these vary from excellent sources such as the Epilepsy Foundation or epilepsy.com to sites of misinformation that can be harmful.

The AAN in their educational efforts have admirably addressed the issue of patient education for many neurological disorders. The topic of epilepsy is here addressed by Ilo Leppik, M.D. Few are as qualified for this task. A senior clinician-epileptologist and clinical investigator, Leppik has long assumed a role in educating a broad audience about epilepsy.

This book takes the reader from understanding of seizures and epilepsy to topics of diagnosis and management. Especially notable is Dr. Leppik's ability to translate complex subjects such as neurotransmission or imaging into descriptions that allow the nonexpert to understand the subject. The discussion of treatment and especially properties of various antiepileptic drugs are covered in detail. Other parts of the volume address more social but very important subjects such as concerns about operation of a motor vehicle and laws that often differ from state to state.

Some of the book covers topics in great detail, but the organization of the chapters allows readers to review topics of primary interest.

Richard H. Mattson, MD
Professor of Neurology
Yale University

Preface

EPILEPSY IS A COMMON DISORDER, but many people understood it poorly. Over the last few decades there have been many improvements in the treatment of epilepsy. The amount of information needed to give the best care is now very large. In an effort to achieve the best possible outcome, it is important for both persons with epilepsy and their supporters to be as informed as possible. This will lead persons with epilepsy to work in close partnership with their health care professionals to get the best medical care as well as to improve other areas of their lives including education, employment, transportation, and leisure activities.

Having had seizures or having seen someone else have seizures can very frightening and can cause great anxiety. The fear is often not necessary. Knowing what epilepsy is, how it is best treated, and what the chances are for leading a normal life will help to decrease worry. This book will help answer many of your concerns and reassure you that what is happening can be helped, and that things will get better. Most persons with epilepsy can lead full, productive, and satisfying lives once they get the proper care and understand the condition better.

WHAT ARE SEIZURES AND WHAT IS EPILEPSY?

A seizure is a short, single event, usually lasting a few seconds and rarely more than a few minutes, during which a person has uncontrollable strange or violent behavior. The smallest seizures may be noticeable only to the person having the seizure. The largest ("grand mal") seizures can be dramatic convulsions with the person falling to the ground unconscious, foaming at the mouth, and shaking violently.

A seizure is the expression of abnormal brain activity during which the normal electrochemical processes are temporarily "short-circuited." Epilepsy is a condition of the brain that leads to more than one seizure.

The brain of a person with epilepsy can be working normally for days, months, or years and then suddenly, often without warning, experience a seizure. After recovery, which may sometimes be instant, or at worst, a day or two, there may again be a long period of normal activity. One way to understand this is to compare the brain to a computer with a circuit that is not wired properly. This computer can perform complicated activities for long periods of time, but then can "crash" unexpectedly and at an inconvenient time. Once it has been restarted, however, it can work well again for long periods of time. Ultimately, it is the uncertainty of when the next seizure will occur that causes much of the fear and limitations that people with epilepsy have to deal with.

One source of confusion associated with epilepsy is that seizures can be triggered by conditions outside of the brain which can cause it to become over-excited. These conditions include low blood sugar, high fever, drugs, heart conditions, or illnesses that cause imbalances in body chemistry. Seizures caused by these conditions are not considered to be epileptic seizures because the brain is being stressed by conditions outside of the brain. They are called "nonepileptic seizures."

To have a diagnosis of epilepsy, a person must have part of the brain trigger a seizure while the rest of the body is normal. Epilepsy can be caused by a number of different things, including head injury, stroke, tumor, infection, and many other medical conditions. However, the exact cause cannot be identified.

A BRIEF HISTORY OF EPILEPSY

Seizures and epilepsy have always been part of the human condition. The earliest known writings on clay tablets from the Mesopotamian civilization (present-day Iraq), which are more than 5,000 years old, have descriptions of behaviors that today would be classified as generalized tonic-clonic seizures, complex partial seizures, and absence seizures. An ancient Greek, Aretaeus, wrote "epilepsy is an illness of various shapes and horrible." Hippocrates, the famous Greek physician, recognized that seizures came from the brain. He used the word *aura*, which means "breeze" in Greek, to describe the feeling a young man had just before his seizure. Some groups believed that convulsions were associated with divine communication, and persons with epilepsy were sometimes used as oracles. On the other hand, some religions considered persons with epilepsy to be possessed by demons or the devil. Because of these mistaken beliefs, many persons with epilepsy have faced great difficulties over the years.

In spite of the limitations of having seizures, many people with epilepsy have had successful careers, and many famous people have had "the falling sickness." Alexander the Great had occasional seizures while conquering the Middle East, India, and Egypt. Julius Caesar sustained some brain damage during a long delivery at birth, and was finally delivered by a procedure now known as a Caesarian section. He tried to keep his epilepsy a secret, but Cleopatra found out about it while spying on him, and she is rumored to have used her knowledge of his epilepsy to her benefit. One of the best descriptions of a seizure was written by Fyodor Dostoevsky, the Russian novelist, who had epilepsy. In his novel, *The Idiot,* he describes an aura as a very strong feeling of pleasure, which he knows will then be followed by a convulsion. Alfred Nobel, founder of the Nobel Prize, had epilepsy. In spite of his epilepsy, he invented dynamite. These are but a few of the many persons who lived at a time when there was no effective treatment for epilepsy. Today, there are many people living with epilepsy whose lives have been greatly improved with the treatments now available.

EPILEPSY TODAY

Epilepsy is a common neurological disorder that affects persons of all ages from newborns to the elderly. At the present time, it is estimated that from 1.5 to 2 million people in the United States have active epilepsy. Many more have had epilepsy at some time in their life. As many as one out of ten persons will have a seizure at some time in their lives, but the majority will not have epilepsy because the convulsions are caused by conditions outside of the brain. Because many people can have seizures without having epilepsy, making the correct diagnosis after a seizure is very important.

Why Is There So Much Confusion About Epilepsy?

Understanding epilepsy can be very confusing, and unless you have a clear framework for making sense of it, many things you hear or read can create misunderstanding. This book will help clarify many of these issues. Epilepsy is not a single disease. Rather, it is a disorder of many causes, types of seizures, and of varying severity. It is difficult to understand because:

- Many attacks that look like seizures may not be seizures.
- Many seizures are not epileptic seizures.
- There are many different types of epileptic seizures.
- There are many causes of epilepsy.
- The severity of epilepsy can range from mild, with only a few seizures during a lifetime, to very severe, with many seizures each week.
- Epilepsy can be present with no other problems, or it can be associated with many other problems with brain functioning.

The first chapter of this book will explain the differences between epileptic and nonepileptic seizures. The second chapter will review the different types of epileptic seizures. The third chapter will discuss the various epilepsy syndromes. And the remaining chapters will discuss treatments and other issues to improve the quality of life for the person with epilepsy.

Suggested Reading

Temkin O. *The Falling Sickness: A History of Epilepsy from the Greeks to the Beginnings of Modern Neurology*, 2nd edition, revised. Baltimore and London, Johns Hopkins Press, 1971.

Hauser WA, Hesdorffer DC, eds: *Epilepsy: Frequency, Causes, and Consequences*. New York, Demos, 1990.

Epilepsy

CHAPTER 1

Diagnosing Epilepsy

T HE ACCURATE DIAGNOSIS OF EPILEPSY can be difficult and confusing. This is because one must consider three possibilities after an event of loss of consciousness or abnormal behavior. First, did the event look like a seizure, but really was a faint or panic attack? Second, was it a seizure caused by conditions outside of the brain, and therefore not epilepsy? Finally, if it was a seizure originating in the brain, will it happen again? A diagnosis of epilepsy should be made only if there is a condition of the brain that will likely lead to additional seizures.

WHAT IS A SEIZURE?

Today, when the term is used medically, seizure means a sudden, unexpected change in a person's behavior that lasts for only a short time—usually no more than a few minutes—caused by a temporary disturbance in brain activity. There are many different types of seizures. Some are only an unusual feeling or sensation. These are called simple partial seizures. Others are a loss of awareness of surroundings, while behaving unusually and having no memory of what happened. These are called complex partial seizures. The most serious seizures, formerly called "grand mal," involve falling to the ground with the whole body jerking (convulsing) for one to two minutes. These seizures may involve tongue biting, urination, and loss of bowel control.

THE FIRST SEIZURE

For persons who have never had a seizure, the first convulsion is a very frightening event. But it can be even more upsetting to people close to them. Persons having a convulsive seizure may or may not have a brief warning. After that, they are unconscious during the seizure and for some time afterward. Their first memory is often of waking up in the ambulance or at the hospital. Depending on the circumstances, they may have had an injury from falling, a bitten tongue, or loss of urine or bowel control. Waking up in these circumstances is very troubling.

The emotional trauma of the spouse, friend, or parent is even more severe because they witnessed the convulsion. If it happens during the day, everything appears to be normal. Then, suddenly, there may be a brief grunt or cry; the person's eyes may be wide open and staring ahead. The jaw will be tightly shut and the body stiff. The legs are often straight and the arms at the side. The person may then fall—usually forward or backward, but hardly ever to the side. On the way down, they may hit furniture or other objects. As they hit the ground, their head may be injured. This is the stiff, or tonic phase of a generalized tonic-clonic ("grand mal") seizure or convulsion. (See Figure 1-1.) During the tonic phase, the chest muscles are contracted, squeezing the lungs and veins returning blood to the heart. This pushes the venous blood, which is blue, into the face making it look cyanotic (blue). Because the person is not breathing, and the face is turning blue, it is natural to panic. The tonic phase may last for 10 to 30 seconds. It is followed by the clonic (jerking) phase during which the muscles relax briefly and the arms relax at the elbow, with the hands coming toward the side of the body. The mouth may open briefly and the tongue may fall between the teeth. This lasts only a second or two, and the arms bend at the elbows and come towards the face and the legs straighten out again. This time, as the

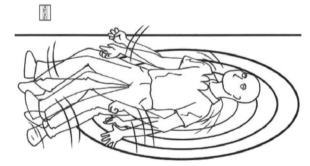

FIGURE 1-1

Generalized tonic-clonic seizure, former-ly called a "grand mal" seizure. The person was helped to lie down on a rug to avoid injury.

jaw clenches (shuts tightly) the side of the tongue may be bitten. The clonic phase may last one or two minutes, with the periods of relaxation increasing at the end. At the end of the tonic-clonic seizure, the person is unconscious and all of the muscles are exhausted and relaxed.

Because the tongue muscles relax, the tongue often falls to the back of the mouth, but the tongue is never swallowed, as is often thought by some people. Because the person did not breathe for the 1 or 2 minutes during the seizure, there is very heavy and deep breathing after the seizure to replenish oxygen. The most important first aid measure is to roll the person to the side so that the tongue can fall to the side of the mouth and not block breathing. In the past, it was believed than an object should be put into the mouth of the person having a seizure. We now know that this is the worst thing one can do because it may block breathing and/or cause the person to vomit. If the person vomits and then breathes, stomach acid can enter the lungs and cause a life-threatening pneumonia. (See Table 1-1 for a full description of proper first aid.)

Usually, after a seizure, the person breathes very deeply for 3 to 4 minutes and additional oxygen is not needed. The person then begins to recover consciousness. After a first seizure, the person seeing the seizure should call for an ambulance.

How Does My Physician Know If I Have Epilepsy?

After a suspected first seizure, a number of important decisions need to be made. Some of the basic decisions relating to acute care will be made in the emergency room. But because epilepsy is a chronic (long-term) condition that can have serious effects on driving, employment, and social relationships, it is important to have a physician expert in the evaluation of seizures and conditions that resemble seizures review the case. (See Figure 1-2.)

Was It a Seizure?

One of the physician's most important tasks in evaluating a patient who has lost consciousness is to determine if the event was a seizure or syn-

3

Table 1-1 First Aid for Seizures

Generalized tonic-clonic seizures
At the onset or during the seizure:
- Help the person lie or sit down
- Remove eyeglasses
- Clear area of harmful objects
- Loosen tight clothing around the neck
- Do not restrain the person
- Do not force any object into the person's mouth

After the seizure:
- Turn the person to one side to permit mouth to drain
- Continue to observe the person until he or she is fully awake

Look for an identifying bracelet. If the person is known to have epilepsy, it is not necessary to call for medical help unless:

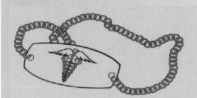

- An injury has occurred
- Seizures do not stop within two or three minutes
- A second seizure occurs
- The person requests an ambulance

Complex partial seizures
The person may stare without focusing, not speak, perform aimless movements, smack lips or appear to chew, fidget with clothes. Sometimes this behavior resembles that of a drunk or drugged person.

During the seizure:
- Do not try to stop or restrain the person
- Guide the person gently away from harmful objects

After the seizure:
- Stay with the person until she or he is fully alert
- Reassure others that this behavior was caused by a medical condition

cope ("fainting, passing out"). Syncopal events are the most common symptoms confused with seizures, especially if there is inadequate history or observational data. Brief clonic activity often accompanies syncope, and this can often lead to confusion regarding the diagnosis. However, the character of the muscle activity in syncope is mostly clonic or myoclonic, involves distal extremities, and rarely causes the classical axial tonic posturing (stiff body) seen in a tonic-clonic seizure.

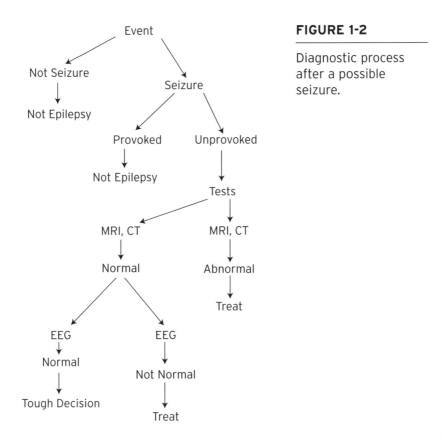

FIGURE 1-2

Diagnostic process after a possible seizure.

There are many causes of syncope, as listed in Table 1-2. For example, a medical student, after donating blood and suffering from sleep deprivation, stood up, became pale, lost consciousness, fell slowly to the ground, had some clonic activity of his hands, and lost bladder control (wet his pants). Although he was initially diagnosed as having had a seizure, the setting of the event and clinical features later led to the more accurate diagnosis of syncope. Strong emotional situations can lead to very rapid breathing and dizziness, vision blanking, and loss of consciousness. After losing consciousness from hyperventilation, a person often will not breathe for a minute or two as the body attempts to restore a normal chemical balance. This is just the opposite of the deep, heavy breathing seen after a generalized tonic-clonic seizure, but it can frighten an onlooker into thinking something life-threatening has happened. Children sometimes play a game where one child will hyperven-

Table 1-2.   Some Conditions That May Be Mistaken for Seizures

1. Syncope (fainting, "passing out")
   Vasovagal attack
   • Hyperventilation-induced syncope
   Cardiac
   • Atrioventricular block
   • Adams-Stokes attack
   • Sinoatrial block
   • Paroxysmal tachycardia
   • Reflex cardiac arrhythmia
   • Other cardiac causes of decreased cardiac output
   Hypovolemia
   Hypotension (sudden drop in blood pressure)
   Micturition syncope
   Cough syncope
2. Nonepileptic seizures of psychogenic origin ("pseudoseizures" or "psychogenic seizures")
3. Breath-holding spells (in children)
4. Paroxysmal REM sleep behavior (violent behavior during sleep)
5. Panic attack

tilate and then another child will wrap his or her arms around the chest and squeeze, causing a vagal reflex, slow heart, and syncope. This is usually harmless, but occasionally will be accompanied by some clonic activity that can be very frightening to a parent.

Cardiogenic syncope is seen most often in older persons who have a heart condition. Feeling for a pulse can be very helpful. After a generalized tonic-clonic seizure the pulse is usually fast, regular, and strong. With cardiogenic syncope, the pulse may be weak and irregular. Cardiac causes of syncope can often be diagnosed by electro-cardiogram (EKG). Micturition syncope (fainting after urination) may be seen in men with prostate problems. Cough syncope may be seen in persons with emphysema who faint after coughing heavily. Both are reflexes involving the vagus nerve and cause slowing of the heart leading to hypotension (low blood pressure), loss of consciousness, falls, and sometimes injury.

Non-epileptic (NEE) seizures of psychogenic origin are often dramatic There is often a great deal of motor activity that is usually considerably more complex than simple tonic-clonic activity. There may be pelvic thrusting, side-to-side head shaking, asynchronous extremity movements, and other embellishments. These often last for many minutes, and sometimes even hours. Because they may be mistaken for status epilepticus (Chapter 11), large doses of medicines may be used. They are often a response to severe emotional stress and often happen to women who have been victims of sexual abuse. Panic attacks may also be misinterpreted as seizures.

PROVOKED SEIZURES

After it has been determined that an episode was a seizure and not syncope, it still does not mean that the person has epilepsy. The seizure may have been provoked, that is, caused by something outside of the brain, thus inducing a change in brain chemistry. A number of medical conditions and lifestyles may provoke seizures (Table 1-3). To determine this, a thorough review of the person's past medical history, use of drugs and other products, social habits, and family history must be done. This may be impossible immediately after the seizure because the patient may be confused, disoriented, or unable or unwilling to disclose sensitive information, such as drug use. In addition, results of the EEG, CT, and MRI scans must be evaluated.

There are many medical conditions that can cause seizures. When a person is brought to the emergency room, a number of tests are done to determine if the seizure was caused by dehydration, abnormal sodi-

Table 1-3 Some Things That May Provoke Seizures	
Street Drugs:	**Natural Products:**
Cocaine (crack)	Ephedra
Methamphetamine (Meth)	Man Hong
PCP (Angel Dust)	Ginko
	Bitter Lemon
Prescription Drugs:	**Life Style:**
Metabolic Stimulants (usually for weight loss)	Binge alcohol use
Antipsycotic drugs (some)	Sleep deprivation
	Use of stimulant containing beverages or pills
Acute Head Trauma:	**Medical Conditions:**
Post-impact seizure	Diabetes
	High fever
	Low oxygen
	Electrolyte imbalance (low sodium)

um level, low potassium level, abnormal blood sugar, pneumonia, kidney failure, liver failure, infections, or other conditions thay may trigger convulsions.

Drugs and natural products that stimulate the brain may cause convulsions. In some regions, the major cause of seizures is the use of street drugs that excite the brain, such as methamphetamine and crack cocaine. Alcohol abuse has for many years been a major cause, and many medical reports have discussed the phenomenon of alcohol withdrawal seizures. Many prescription and non-prescription weight-loss products have the potential for causing convulsions. Most of these promise to "speed up metabolism," "burn up calories," and other similar claims, but they over-stimulate the brain.

Many over-the-counter drugs containing stimulants have been withdrawn by the Food and Drug Administration (FDA). However, this agency has no regulatory power over "natural products." Because of this, natural products do not need to be tested for safety. Unfortunately, some heavily marketed products contain substances that are strong stimulants, and there are many reports in the medical literature about people who have had seizures after using products that contain ephedra, *mau hong*, bitter lemon, gingko, and others. Most hospital emergency departments can test urine or blood for these compounds in a group of tests called the tox battery (short for toxicology battery). If the seizure was provoked by one of these substances, simply not using them will avoid future seizures and the person should not be diagnosed as having epilepsy.

Another common situation in which seizures happen occurs on college campuses. College life can provide many situations that can be stressful to the brain. One common story is that a student had a convulsion, and all of the testing was normal. The worry was that this was epilepsy. But reviewing the details of events two days before the seizure revealed that there was an upcoming examination, the student used highly caffeinated beverages or readily available "keep awake" pills, missed lots of sleep, and then had a convulsion. Or, the student partied for many hours, consumed alcohol, may have used other substances, missed sleep, and then the next morning, often while still asleep, had a convulsion. These students should be diagnosed as having had a provoked seizure and not given a diagnosis of epilepsy. Rather, a diagnostic code of "convulsion not otherwise specified" is used.

Stimulants can cause seizures at the time of use while measurable amounts of the drugs are still in the body. However, many drugs commonly used for anxiety, if used heavily, can cause withdrawal seizures that occur some days after the last dose. For example, a woman from the Twin Cities travelled to Arizona to visit relatives. A few days after arriving, she had two generalized tonic-clonic seizures in one day. She was told she had epilepsy and was started on antiepileptic medications. Upon returning, she was re-evaluated, and only after a thorough review of events surrounding the seizure did she reveal that she had been a heavy user of benzodiazepines for sleep and anxiety, and had forgotten to take her medications to Arizona. In retrospect, she had seizures provoked by benzodiazepine withdrawal. The antiepileptic drugs she had been treated with were slowly withdrawn, and the diagnosis of epilepsy was reversed.

A common condition in sports with body contact is the post-impact seizure. An example of this was seen on TV some years ago when a football quarterback had a convulsion after being sacked. He was taken to the hospital where no serious injuries were found. He was not treated and continued playing. An Australian research team studied the outcomes of hundreds of soccer players who had a post-impact convulsion documented on video and found that their risk for developing epilepsy was no different than for the general population. However, a seizure occurring 24 hours or later after a head injury may be a sign that epilepsy may develop.

All of these people have had a provoked seizure. They should not be diagnosed as having epilepsy, and will usually not have another seizure if they avoid the behaviors that provoked the initial seizures or are treated for the medical condition. In a few cases, however, they may have seizures later on that were not provoked and the issue of epilepsy being present needs to be re-evaluated.

Unprovoked Seizures

A more difficult situation is that of a person who has had a seizure, but no provoking factors can be identified. Today, most people who have a seizure have a CT scan and/or MRI scan and an electroencephalogram (EEG) done if no obvious provoking factors are immediately known. Even if a provoking factor is present, these tests may be done to be certain that a brain tumor or previously undiscovered epileptic syndrome is not present. If the CT scan, MRI scan, or EEGs are abnormal and indicate a disorder of the brain likely to lead to more seizures, a diagnosis of epilepsy can be made and appropriate treatment started.

A very common situation, however, is that all of the tests register normal.

The medical definition of epilepsy is usually considered to be two or more seizures. Thus, a person who has had only one seizure and does not have an identifiable brain lesion known to be associated with seizures is in a difficult diagnostic and treatment situation. An unprovoked seizure is clearly an indication that the person has a brain that is more likely than average to have a seizure. But will there be another seizure? Studies have been conducted to answer this question, and have found that of adults who have had a single unprovoked seizure, from 34% to 71% will have a second seizure. The period of time between the first and the second seizure can be many years, but during the first two years is the most likely period. Also, looking at these statistics in reverse, we can say that 29% to 66% will not have another seizure. One large, long-term study of 208 teenagers and adults with one unprovoked seizure found that overall 34% of the study participants had had a second seizure within 5 years of their first seizure. Ten percent had their second seizure within the first year, and 24% had their second seizure at the end of the second year. Thus, most people who will have more seizures will have their second one within two years of their first event.

This study also found that one very important risk factor for having more seizures was having siblings (brothers or sisters) with epilepsy. Most of the patients in the study did not have a sibling with epilepsy. However, among those who had a sibling with epilepsy, the recurrence rate was 29% after one year and 46% after five years following the first seizure. Having a parent or grandparent increased the risk but not by much. Because seizures happen to approximately 11% of all people during their lifetime (approximately one in 10), having two or three relatives out of 20 relatives with seizures is not uncommon, so having a relative such as a cousin with epilepsy is not uncommon and does not seem to greatly increase the risk.

Another risk factor was having seizures with fever or other illness. Thus, while most persons with a febrile convulsion in childhood do not have seizures later in life, many people who have a seizure later in life will have had a febrile or provoked seizure earlier. Persons who had a previous history of head trauma, stroke, meningitis, cerebral palsy, or other brain injury also had a higher risk for a second seizure. Another risk factor for additional seizures was the presence of a specific EEG finding. Thus, a person with a single unprovoked seizure with any of the risk factors listed would seriously need to consider starting treatment to prevent additional seizures.

A more difficult decision arises for those patients with none of the additional risk factors. For these patients, the probability of a second seizure is less than 10% in the first year and approximately 24% by the end of two years after the single seizure. Is this a high enough rate to warrant the risks of treatment? There is no single answer to this question. The decision to treat or not to treat must be based on an evaluation by the patient and physician of the risks and benefits. As described in Chapter 4, the risk of treatment with available antiepileptic medications is generally low. The impact of a second seizure depends on the patient's lifestyle. Treatment may be indicated for patients needing to drive, or for those who face significant risk of injury or loss of self-esteem from a second seizure. The risk of recurrence is greatest in the first two years, so if treatment is started, it probably can be discontinued after the highest risk period passes.

Treatment is based on the assumption that recurrent seizures can be prevented with adequate medication. Only a few studies have examined treatment after a single seizure. One study randomized (chosen by chance) half of 397 patients aged 2 to 70 years to receive treatment with an antiepileptic drug after a single unprovoked generalized tonic-clonic seizure, and the other half to receive a placebo (inactive pill). The treatment group had a risk of seizure recurrence of about half of those not treated. Thus, limited clinical studies and intuition would suggest that treatment may prevent some but not all persons from having additional seizures if treated after a single unprovoked seizure.

In considering the issue of when to treat, social factors must be taken into account. For an adult, the most important question is whether this should affect the person's ability to drive a motor vehicle. In most states, a single seizure is not always considered grounds for restricting driving, but the presence of epilepsy as demonstrated by the occurrence of two or more seizures subjects the patient to numerous restrictions. Some patients, after reviewing the odds with their physician, elect to begin treatment after a single seizure. These decisions are difficult and should never be made unilaterally by the physician for the patient. Rather, the patient should be aware of the risks and benefits of the alternative strategies. In children, there may be less pressure to treat and the side-effects profile may be less beneficial than in adults. Also, identification of a specific epilepsy syndrome can be useful in deciding whether to treat. The risk of a third seizure after a second unprovoked seizure is approximately 75%, so there is no debate about treating after a second seizure.

What Is an EEG?

Unlike the CT or MRI scan, which show the structure, or anatomy, of the brain, an EEG shows the electrical activity of the brain. The information it provides is entirely different from information obtained from structural studies. To give an example, at the time of death, electrical activity of the brain and heart will be absent (flat line EEG or EKG), but a CT scan of the brain or heart may be normal.

The EEG detects very small electrical signals generated by the brain, which are detectable from the scalp by using very sensitive recording equipment. These signals are only a few millionths of a volt. It would take about 500,000 people standing in a line with their heads wired up to generate the same voltage as a flashlight battery. To record an EEG, a person must have electrical contacts placed on the head. These must be placed firmly so they do not move and disturb the recording. Many EEG laboratories use a special kind of strong, quick-drying glue. The contacts

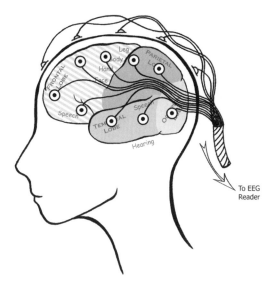

FIGURE 1-3

Placement of EEG electrodes over specific areas of the brain to help locate the region from which seizures are starting.

To EEG Reader

are placed on locations determined by careful measurement so the contacts are over specific parts of the brain (Figure 1-3). The physician interpreting the record can therefore determine from what part the abnormal activity is coming. Most laboratories now process the EEG signals digitally. Until recently, they were recorded on paper. Many laboratories also record an EKG at the same time to make sure that abnormalities seen on an EEG are not coming from the heart. Also, because some seizures arise from cardiac arrythmias (irregular heart beat), it is useful to get more information from the heart. EEGs can be recorded for as little as 30 minutes and up to 6 hours in a medical office. They can also be recorded continuously in the hospital using video cameras at the same time to capture seizures (video-EEG).

The background rhythm of a normal, waking EEG consists of alpha activity of 20 to 50 microvolts (20 to 50 millionths of a volt). This activity is less than one-hundredth of the amplitude of cardiac potentials. Thus, the EEG signals are much more difficult to detect, and with DC amplifiers the EEG signals would be completely masked by muscle and cardiac activity. However, the development of AC amplifiers and bipolar recording has made it possible to measure the small, brain-generated potentials. Still, it should be obvious that in the presence of many rela-

13

tively higher physiologic potentials, the EEG is subject to a great deal of artifact (stray signals not from the brain). Indeed, the most difficult aspect of EEG interpretation is correctly recognizing artifacts and not misinterpreting them as pathological. Many mistakes have been made in diagnosing the presence of epilepsy when the abnormality was later determined to be an artifact. Guidelines have been established for the proper technical qualifications for EEG laboratories and technicians. There are specialty boards for physicians who specialize in interpreting EEGs.

An EEG requires the placement of 21 standard electrodes over the scalp. Additional electrodes, such as sphenoidal electrodes that are inserted under the skin at the upper edge of the jawbone, may be used in some cases. The EEG electrodes are connected to the amplifiers in pairs. These can be linked up in a number of ways. Many EEG machines have 16 channels. These are recorded simultaneously because it is necessary to be able to develop a "map" of abnormal activity. In addition, because seizures may in some instances be triggered by hyperventilation or photic stimulation, these activation techniques should be performed in all EEGs.

A major problem in the diagnosis of epilepsy is that the EEG may be normal for long periods relative to the time of the recording. Epileptiform activity may be present only for a few seconds sometimes hours apart. It is not uncommon for a standard 30-minute recording to show no definite interictal activity (activity that indicates an abnormality associated with epilepsy but comes between seizures) in the presence of diagnosed epilepsy. Studies have shown that only 50% to 60% of routine EEGs (30 minutes, no sleep deprivation) obtained after a seizure in patients later clearly diagnosed as having epilepsy show epileptiform abnormalities.

While normal EEGs are not useful, abnormal recordings are very helpful. Two things can be learned from the EEG. The first is determination of the presence of epilepsy. The finding of an epileptiform EEG and the history of a seizure are strong evidence of the existence of a brain disorder associated with a risk for further seizures. The second major purpose of the EEG is the classification of the epilepsy as localization-related or generalized. In addition, the localization of the discharge is helpful in determining the area of the brain containing the epileptogenic lesion (Figure 1-3). Knowledge of the probable site of origin can help guide other diagnostic studies.

The signature of an epileptic EEG abnormality is the sharp transient (a sudden change in voltage), which is usually a spike (less than 80 milliseconds—thousandths of a second) or a sharp wave. A number of computer programs have been developed for spike detection, but for clinical diagnosis visual interpretation is still needed to screen out artifacts (stray signals). Spikes may be focal or generalized. Muscle artifact, EKG potential, movement artifacts, and "electrode pops" must be differentiated from activity of central nervous system (brain) origin.

One of the most common errors made is the misreading of EKG potential or other sharp activity as spikes. In the intensive care unit, even the electromagnetic field generated by a drop of saline (salt water) from an intravenous drip may be recorded and appear as a spike. In addition, there are many CNS (central nervous system) signals such as small sharp spikes, 14 and 6 spike-and-wave complexes, and other phenomena that may be misinterpreted as abnormal but are variations of normal activity brain in some patients. An example of EEG seizure activity is shown in Figure 1-4.

WHAT IS A CT SCAN?

A computed tomography (CT) scan, or sometimes called computed axial tomography (CAT) scan, is in fact a very sophisticated X-ray. In conventional X-rays, the subject is placed between a source of X-rays and a photographic film (Figure 1-5). Only one picture can be taken for each film plate, and the physician gets only one two-dimensional picture. With a CT scanner, the patient lies within a large circular scanner that has an X-ray source and a detector mounted on it. The scanner revolves around the patient and takes many images, each at a different angle. Instead of film, the CT scanner uses a detector that records digital data that is sent to a computer, similar to how a digital camera works (Figure 1-6). The computer then reconstructs the information into a three-dimensional data set, which is then viewed on a computer screen or

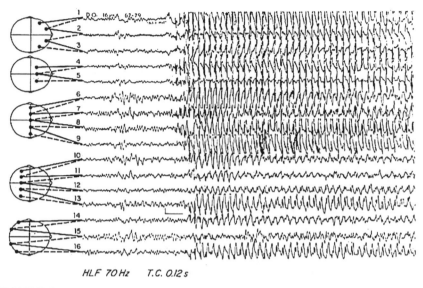

HLF 70 Hz   T.C. 0.12 s

FIGURE 1-4

EEG showing normal brain activity for the first few seconds, replaced by generalized seizure activity for the rest of the sample.

made into a series of pictures on standard X-ray film. A CT scan, like an X-ray, shows how much of the X-ray is absorbed by the various tissues.

Tissue that contains elements of higher atomic weight, such as calcium or iron, absorb more X-rays than tissues that contain lower atomic

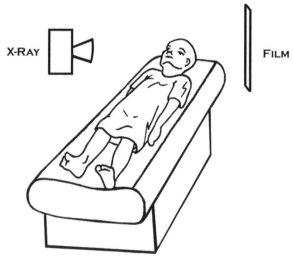

X-RAY

FILM

FIGURE 1-5

A conventional X-ray machine with a beam generated by the X-ray tube passing through the patient, with film recording the amount not blocked by the subject. Bone absorbs more X-rays than tissue and looks white on the picture.

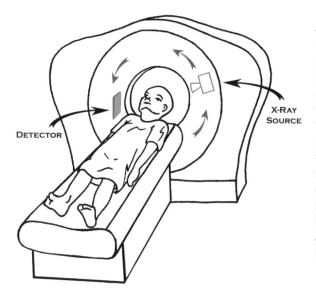

DETECTOR

X-RAY
SOURCE

FIGURE 1-6

CT scanner. An X-ray source and a detector are mounted at opposite ends of a wheel, which turns around the head. This allows many angles of view that can display the skull and brain in three dimensions. An MRI scanner looks similar, but uses radio signals and magnetic fields instead of X-rays.

weight elements, such as carbon. Substances containing hydrogen, such as water, absorb the least. Bone, high in calcium, absorbs many X-rays and looks white, whereas brain tissue absorbs less and looks darker.

Thus, the CT scan is much better than a single X-ray on film, but basically highlights the same findings. The CT scan is able to show slices of the brain to the physician, allowing much more detail to be seen, and also is able to show tissues within the brain better than an X-ray. Like a conventional X-ray, the CT scan exposes the subject to potentially damaging X-rays. However, the exposure is low and the risk is very small and it should be considered in light of its benefits and other risks. It has been estimated that one cross-Atlantic round trip flight has the same radiation exposure as a CT scan of the head. CT scans are readily available in hospitals now and are very useful for detecting bleeding in the brain and many large tumors.

WHAT IS AN MRI SCAN?

A magnetic resonance imaging (MRI) scan uses a property of tissues that is entirely different from X-rays. All chemical bonds (the forces that hold atoms together to form molecules, which form tissues) "vibrate" or resonate at specific frequencies based on their elements. Thus, water with hydrogen bonds will have a different resonance pattern than fat or bone. In an MRI machine, a very strong magnetic field (strong enough to wipe out the information on a credit card or pull a screw out of an object in the room) is set up to hold the molecules in line while radio waves of certain frequencies are passed through the body. Detectors pick up the signals generated and, as with a CT scan, convert them into computer displays or print them on film. Information can also be put on to a CD so a physician or technician can carry them. Information can also be transmitted through the Internet to the offices of different physicians. Sometimes scans are even sent to other hospitals or other countries to be interpreted.

Although a CT scan and MRI scan look similar, they show tissues differently. A CT scan is more sensitive to blood and bone, whereas the MRI can show tissue differences too subtle for the CT. This is especially true for some brain tumors. In general, the CT is a good scan for emergencies, especially if there has been trauma, while an MRI is much better at diagnosing tumors (see Figure 1-7), abnormal brain tissue patterns, and changes such as mesial temporal sclerosis. Another advantage of the MRI is that there is no exposure to radiation. However, because

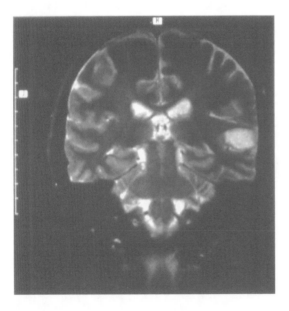

FIGURE 1-7

A brain tumor detected by an MRI but missed by a CT scan. Can you find the tumor?
(The answer is on p. 153 in Appendix 1.)

Table 1-4 How EEG, CT, and MRI Differ

EEG	CT	MRI
Records the electrical activity of the brain.	Uses X-rays to show brain structure.	Uses magnetic field and radio frequency waves to show brain structure.
Can detect circuit changes even when MRI and CT are normal	Best for tissues with bone and blood.	Best for changes in gray and white matter and small structural changes.
Helps classify epilepsy syndrome and locate focal seizures are generated.	Useful after head injury and screening for tumors and vascular malformations.	Best for locating slow-growing tumors, diagnosing mesial temporal sclerosis and cortical heterotopias.
Basic concepts developed in 1920, computerized data processing has replaced paper recording.	Concepts of X-rays developed early 1900's, computer analysis has permitted more detail and 3 dimensional analysis.	Basic concepts developed in 1950s; application to medicine began in mid-1980s.

of the strong magnetic field, people who have iron or other magnetic metals in their body cannot have an MRI. Many surgeons now use metal clips made of materials that can be used in an MRI. Amalgam dental fillings are safe in an MRI, as are lead bullets, but not steel fragments. Before you have an MRI, you should tell the doctor and technician about any possible metal you may have in your body from previous surgeries, battles, or incidents.

Table 1-4 compares some of the features of EEG, CT, and MRI scans.

CHAPTER 2

Types of Seizures

How Does the Brain Work?

B EFORE WE BEGIN TO DISCUSS the different types of seizures, epileptic syndromes, medicines, and surgical treatments available, it is useful to understand the basic concepts on how the brain works.

Our brain controls all of our activities—walking, talking, seeing, hearing, smelling, feeling, and so on. The brain is an electrochemical organ that has billions of nerve cells (neurons) connected by axons and dendrites (biological wires) to other neurons or action cells such as muscle cells or glands. When the brain is working normally, all of our actions follow patterns that can be anticipated and controlled. The place where a neuron touches another neuron, or action cell, is called a *synapse*. A synapse contains small packets of chemicals that are released when a neuron is electrically excited (Figures 2-1 and 2-2). These chemicals travel to the membrane (skin) of the other cell and cause a small electrical current by opening pores to let in charged atoms (sodium, chloride, calcium, or potassium).

Depending upon the kind of cell that is releasing the packet, the receiving cell can be either excited or depressed. If the receiving neuron, which receives signals from hundreds or thousands of other neurons, receives enough excitatory signals, it also becomes excited and releases chemical packets to all of the neurons or action cells to which it is connected. On the other hand, if it receives more depressing (inhibitory) signals, it will not become excited. Normally, neurons in the brain exist in a balance between those that are excitatory (causing actions to take place) and those that are inhibitory (slowing down actions to keep them from going out of control). Seizures happen when too many neurons become

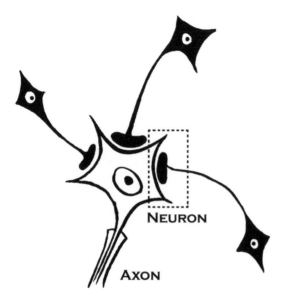

FIGURE 2-1

A diagram of a nerve cell (neuron) and its connections. The dotted line shows Figure 2-2.

NEURON

AXON

excited and start sending abnormal signals to the neurons and muscles, causing behaviors to become abnormal. Meanwhile, inhibitory neurons are trying to restore order. A seizure ends when the excited neurons run out of energy or when enough inhibitory neurons become active.

Normal neurons can start sending abnormal patterns if they lack oxygen or sugar (glucose), or if they are over-stimulated by drugs such as cocaine. Because these seizures are caused by factors outside of the

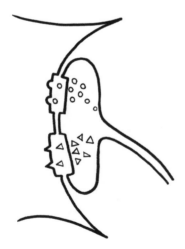

FIGURE 2-2

Enlargement of Figure 2-1 showing a synapse and movement of packets of chemicals.

brain, they are labeled as provoked, or *non-epileptic physiologic* seizures. Sometimes persons have patterns of behavior related to severe psychological stress, but the firing pattern of the neurons is normal. These kinds of seizures are labeled as *non-epileptic psychogenic* seizures. Epileptic seizures, on the other hand, arise from neurons that are damaged or are genetically abnormal.

The major features of seizures that distinguish them from usual activity are that they are stereotypical and repetitive. In addition, they lack the typical behavioral modulations observed in voluntary behavior. For example, a *clonic* seizure involves maximal contraction of skeletal muscles, followed by relaxation, with the cycle usually repeating itself every few seconds. This very primitive pattern of movement accomplishes no useful function and is in marked contrast to the usual complex, modulated activity that our muscles are capable of performing. In short, behaviors during seizures are less complex than normal behavior, and persons cannot carry out activities that require foresight and planning during a seizure.

How Is the Brain Organized?

Much of our present understanding of how the brain is organized was pioneered by Wilder Penfield and his colleagues. He found that the brain is a very highly structured organ with each function located in a very specific area. These discoveries were made during surgery for epilepsy beginning in the 1930s. It is possible to operate on the brain without general anesthesia because the human brain does not feel pain. The neurons are used to located and interpret pain from other parts of the body. Headaches are not brain "pain"; rather, they arise from blood vessels and the membrane around the brain. With local anesthesia, one can block the pain nerves and cut through skin, bone, and brain coverings. It is then possible to map the brain by giving small electrical stimulations to different parts of the brain. These are experienced by the patient as feeling in the finger, movement of a foot, hearing a sound, seeing colors, and so on. (See Figure 2-3.)

By mapping the brain, Dr. Penfield and others found that it was possible to locate which parts of the brain did what and where the damage

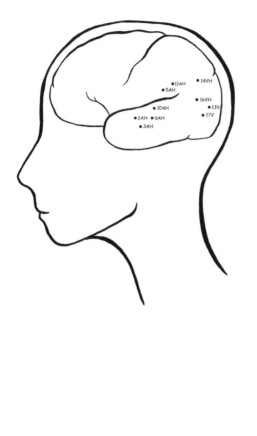

FIGURE 2-3

This patient had electrical stimulation at the points shown by Dr. Wilder Penfield (see reference 1) during surgery under local anesthesia many years ago. She reported seeing colored stars when stimulated at 13V and 17V. When stimulated at 2AH, 3AH, and 6AH she reported hearing memories of her family. These studies show how highly organized the brain is. 13V and 17V are in the occipital lobe where vision is interpreted and 6AH, 2AH, and 3AH are in the temporal lobe where verbal memory is.

causing the seizures was. Then it was possible to carefully remove the part of the brain from which the seizures were originating.

Figure 2-3 was drawn based upon reports given by a patient who was awake during brain surgery for epilepsy. Each spot was a place where a small electrical pulse was given and the patient reported what she experienced. The areas that, when stimulated, reproduced her seizures were removed. Today, epilepsy surgery is done with the patient under general anesthesia, because brain mapping is done as part of an evaluation prior to surgery for epilepsy.

Although the experience gained from surgery for epilepsy was published in 1954, it is still very interesting to read because Dr. Penfield describes what the patients experienced in their own words.

Types of Seizures

Seizures may involve the entire brain or only parts of it. Seizures that involve the entire brain are called generalized seizures, and those that involve only part of the brain are called partial seizures. However, partial seizures can start in one part of the brain and spread to involve the entire brain. Most seizures in adults are partial seizures that spread to involve the entire brain and become generalized tonic-clonic seizures. It is usually the generalized tonic-clonic seizure that gets attention and is identified as the first seizure. However, with careful review of the person's history, in retrospect, unrecognized partial seizures may be found to be present for some time before the generalized tonic-clonic seizure. The most widely accepted way of classifying seizures today was developed during the 1970s as epilepsy specialists recognized how closely the structure of the brain and seizure patterns are related (Table 2-1).

Simple Partial Seizures

Patients with partial seizures rarely make their way to the medical system for assistance. Instead, they are often brought to the hospital emergency department only after an unrecognized and untreated partial seizure generalizes and the patient experiences a generalized tonic-clonic ("grand mal") seizure. The first five symptoms a patient experiences can be a clue to the part of the brain where the seizure starts (Figure 2-4). Most generalized tonic-clonic seizures in adults are secondarily generalized as classified as 1C in Table 2-1. An example of this is a type of seizure called a "Jacksonian seizure," named after a famous neurologist of the nineteenth century. He described patients who would have a seizure that started with thumb jerking, then hand jerking, then face jerking, and finally a generalized tonic-clonic seizure. (See Figures 2-4 and 2-5.) These patients were found to have a lesion in the brain in the area that controls motor activity in the hand opposite the side of the seizures (hence our concept of the right side of the brain controlling the left side of the body, and vice versa). Today we would classify this as a type 1A,1 (simple partial seizure with motor signs) evolving to 1C (partial seizure to secondarily generalized seizure).

Table 2-1 Epileptic Seizures: Classification and Characteristics as Proposed by the International League Against Epilepsy

I. Partial seizures (focal seizures)
  A. Simple partial seizures
    1. with motor signs
    2. with somatosensory or special sensory symptoms
    3. with autonomic symptoms
    4. with psychic symptoms
  B. Complex partial seizures
    1. simple partial onset followed by impairment of consciousness
    2. with impairment of consciousness at the onset
  C. Partial seizures evolving to secondarily generalized seizures
    1. simple partial seizures
        (a) evolving to generalized seizures
    2. complex partial seizures
        (a) evolving to generalized seizures
    3. simple partial seizures evolving to complex partial seizures evolving to generalized seizures

II. Generalized seizures (convulsive or nonconvulsive)
  A. 1. typical absence seizures (petit mal)
      2. atypical
  B. Myoclonic seizures
  C. Clonic seizures
  D. Tonic seizures
  E. Tonic-clonic seizures (grand mal)
  F. Atonic seizures

III. Unclassified epileptic syndromes
  Includes all those seizures that cannot be classified because of incomplete data or because they defy classification into the above categories; for example, neonatal seizures with swimming movements.

IV. Status Epilepticus

(Modified from, *Epilepsia* 1981;22:489-501)

Partial seizures are further subdivided by their effect on consciousness. Seizures in which consciousness is not altered are termed *simple* (Table 2-1, 1A). (See Figure 2-6.) An example of a simple partial seizure is a feeling such as that of a breeze over an extremity. "Aura" is the original Greek word for breeze, and was described in the medical writings of Hippocrates as the sensation felt by a young man just before he was stricken with a generalized tonic-clonic seizure. We now know that the origin of this kind of seizure is in the somatosensory area of the brain,

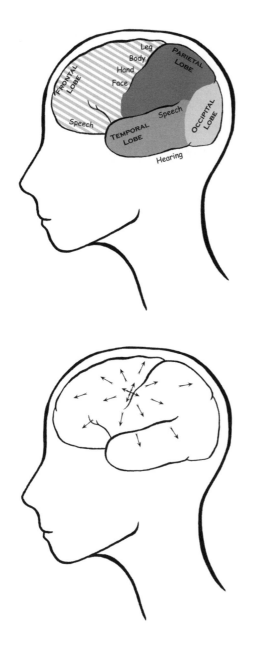

FIGURE 2-4

Organization of the brain into the frontal, parietal, temporal, and occipital lobes. Movement of leg, body, hand, and face are controlled by neurons at the back end of the frontal lobe. Speech is usually on the left side of the brain, in both the frontal lobe and temporal lobe, but these areas provide different speech functions.

FIGURE 2-5

Partial seizure starting in the face and hand motor area of the brain and spreading (generalizes).

contralateral (opposite) to the limb experiencing the feeling. This simple partial seizure may progress into a secondarily generalized tonic-clonic seizure. Using the old terminology, this patient would be described as having an "aura" following by a "grand mal" seizure. (See Figure 2-7.)

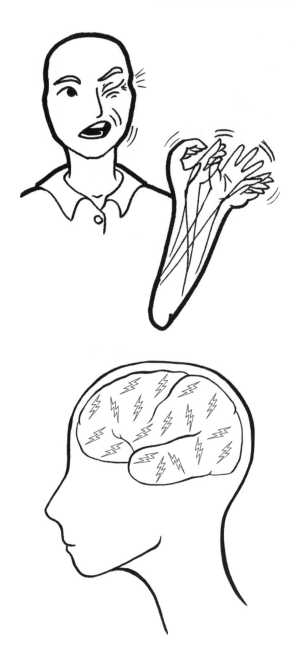

FIGURE 2-6

Simple partial seizure involving the left hand and side of the face. This indicates that the epileptic lesion is located on the right side of the brain in the area shown in Figure 2-3.

FIGURE 2-7

Generalized seizure. The entire brain is involved with the seizure at the beginning.

Seizure manifestations change with medical treatment, so that often a person with Jacksonian seizures may no longer experience generalized tonic-clonic seizures after treatment, but may still have brief motor seizures.

Simple motor seizures (1A,1) arise from the *motor cortex* (frontal lobe) (Figure 2-4). Usually, they consist of rapid clonic activity, but they may be *postural movements* (holding the body in a certain position, such as arm bent at the elbow). Simple partial seizures may exhibit phenomena of various kinds: somatosensory (feeling of a breeze), visual (light flashes, formed visual hallucinations), visual distortions such as macropsia (things appear large), auditory (buzzing), olfactory (a very bad smell), gustatory (a very bad taste), and vertiginous (dizzy feeling or spinning sensation) symptoms. Autonomic symptoms include epigastric rising sensation (described by some as the feeling one gets going down a roller coaster), sweating, flushing, piloerection (goosebumps), and pupillary dilation (the center black part of the eye becomes larger). Psychic symptoms include fear, anger, dreamy states, and the classic *déjà vu* ("I've seen this before") sensation.

Simple partial seizures are sometimes difficult to separate from psychological phenomena. The two key features of epileptic seizures that distinguish them from the manifestations of psychiatric disorders are: (1) seizures occur *paroxysmally* (i.e, without warning and without preceding provocative events); and (2) seizures occur in patients who are relatively free of significant psychiatric disorders. Also of help is the fact that most simple partial seizures last less than a minute. Sometimes, however, it can be difficult to determine whether a patient has had a panic attack or has had a simple, partial psychic seizure. In either case, an accurate diagnosis is needed because the treatments are quite different.

COMPLEX PARTIAL SEIZURES

Complex partial seizures involve impairment, or loss of consciousness. Loss or alteration of consciousness in epilepsy does not refer to coma; rather, a lack of understanding and memory of the event is implied. As Penfield explained, "The state in which an individual is able to move about in a relatively normal manner but is, at the same time, suddenly lacking in understanding is called automatism. Subsequently, (he) will have amnesia (no memory) for the period. He may seem to be an automaton (robot-like) and yet is sometimes partially receptive of direction from others." This implies alteration of functioning in the *mesial temporal* lobes, in the *orbit frontal* lobes, or in more widespread areas of the brain. Complex partial seizures in the past have been referred to as "psychomotor seizures," but this term is vague and ill-defined. And although they have been called "temporal lobe seizures," they can originate from structures other than the temporal lobe.

Complex partial seizures may last a few seconds. These brief episodes may be confused with absence seizures, and sometimes may be called "petit mal." A clear distinction must be made. however, because medications used for absence seizures are not effective for complex partial seizures. Most complex partial seizures last from 1 to 3 minutes, sometimes longer. Patients usually experience a period of confusion after the seizure, lasting for a few minutes. Patients cannot recall any of the events that occurred during the seizure.

The *automatism* (robot-like behavior) has no value in helping to decide on which side of the brain the seizure has started. For example, one right-handed patient snapped his fingers during an automatism, yet his focus was in the right temporal lobe. Sometimes complicated behaviors occur during a complex partial seizure. These often involve partial undressing, urination, or other socially embarrassing behavior, which the patient with epilepsy does not recall after the seizure. "Cursive epilepsy," characterized by frantic running, and "gelastic epilepsy," characterized by uncontrollable laughing, are complex seizures and are classified under 1B,1 or 1 B,2 (Table 2-1), depending on how they started.

Primary Generalized Seizures

Primary generalized seizures involve the entire brain from the outset (Figure 2-7). They can be absence (eye blinking), myclonic, just tonic-, just clonic, tonic-clonic, or atonic. Tonic-clonic seizures are the most dramatic of all seizure types. Generalized tonic-clonic seizures begin suddenly, without warning. (If the patient reports an "aura," the event was most likely a partial seizure with secondary generalization). Typically, the patient cries out as tonic contraction of the trunk muscles forces air out of the lungs. The generalized tonic phase then becomes interrupted by short periods of relaxation followed by tonic contractions.

Then the periods of relaxation become more frequent and the clonic phase begins. The seizure is accompanied by a marked increase in heart rate and blood pressure (Figure 2-8). The seizures last 1 to 2 minutes. After the seizure is over, incontinence may occur as the sphincter muscles relax (not all tonic-clonic seizures are accompanied by incontinence). Full consciousness might not return for 10 to 15 minutes, and confusion and fatigue may persist for hours or days.

Absence seizures are most common in childhood. They are manifested by impairment of consciousness, eye blinking, staring, and other minor facial movements. They last from a few seconds to a minute. However, they may occur many times a day in rapid succession. An important consequence is the time lost, with the result that many children often have poor school performance.

Myoclonic seizures consist of quick muscle jerks. These may be bilateral or unilateral and are usually seen in specific epilepsy syndromes. Consciousness is not usually impaired. However, myoclonic activity may also be associated with other neurologic disorders (Creutzfeldt–Jakob disease, anoxia). Furthermore, it may be difficult to readily categorize myoclonus.

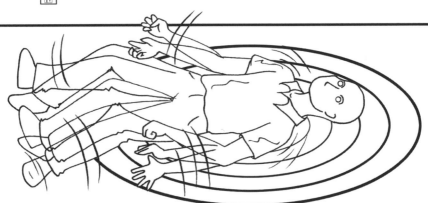

FIGURE 2-8

Generalized tonic-clonic seizure. Patient was helped to lie down on the rug. Eyes are usually open but may be blinking.

Tonic-clonic seizures are the most dramatic seizures and start out with the body being stiff (tonic) and then shaking (clonic) (Figure 2-8). They are the most common seizures causing admission to emergency rooms.

Tonic seizures consist of tonic "spasm" of truncal and facial muscles associated with flexion (bending at the elbows) of upper extremities and extension (straightening at the hips and knees) of lower extremities. They are most common in childhood and may result in falls. They are usually short, lasting only a few seconds.

Clonic seizures are most common in children and may resemble myoclonus, except that there is a loss of consciousness and the repetition rate is slower than in myoclonus.

Atonic seizures are just the opposite of tonic, where all muscles relax and the patient suddenly drops to the floor from a loss of tone in postural muscles. Atonic seizures are most commonly seen in persons with severe damage to both sides of the brain. The attacks generally last only a few seconds and can occur without any loss of consciousness. These seizures are dangerous, however, because they have a high rate of injury from falls. It is often difficult to tell the difference between atonic and tonic seizures.

Suggested Reading

1. Penfield W, Jasper H. *Epilepsy and the Functional Anatomy of the Human Brain*. Boston, Little, Brown and Co., 1954.
2. Commission on Classification and Terminology of the International League Against Epilepsy. Proposal for revised clinical and electroencephalographic classification of epileptic seizures. *Epilepsia* 1981;22:489–501.

CHAPTER 3

Epilepsy and the Epileptic Syndromes

THERE ARE MANY CAUSES of epilepsy. Anything within the brain that alters normal functioning can lead to epilepsy. "Syndrome" is the term used to describe a collection of symptoms and findings from tests that identify a disease. The best treatment can only be given after the specific syndrome is diagnosed. Frequent causes of unsuccessful treatment are not making the correct diagnosis or not using the best drug or, if appropriate, surgery.

The first step in identifying the epileptic syndrome is to identify correctly the type of seizure that a person has had. An epileptic syndrome may include more than one type of seizure. For example, a patient can have both *simple partial motor* and secondarily *generalized tonic-clonic* seizures (types I.A.1 and I.C), but only one syndrome, such as a small tumor near the motor area. Or, a person with the syndrome of juvenile *myoclonic* epilepsy may have *absence*, *myoclonic*, and *generalized tonic-clonic* seizures (types II.A.1, II.B, and II.E). Consequently, a number of pieces of information must be gathered to identify a patient's epileptic syndrome (Table 3-1).

The most important division for identifying the epileptic syndrome is between the *localization-related* epilepsies and the *generalized* epilepsies. A person with localization-related epilepsy has an area of abnormal or damaged neurons that can serve as the starting point for partial seizures. Persons with localization-related epilepsies can be treated with medicines that block the spread of seizure activity, and they may be helped by surgery. Persons with generalized epilepsy usually have a genetically determined abnormality resulting from the way the neurons are built. Some medicines that work for localization-related epilepsies may make

33

Table 3-1 Factors in Identifying the Epileptic Syndrome

- Seizure type(s)
- EEG (ictal and interictal)
- MRI scan
- Response to antiepileptic drugs
- Inheritance

seizures worse in a person with generalized epilepsy, and surgery is not possible for these.

Localization-related epilepsies are described as either *symptomatic* or *cryptogenic*. Symptomatic localization-related epilepsies are the most common syndrome in adults and have many specific identifiable causes (Table 3-2). Despite the large number of causes in this category, seizure types are limited to partial seizures that often, if untreated, progress to secondarily generalized tonic-clonic seizures. The type of seizure is useful in helping decide if it was localization-related, but it is not helpful in identifying the *etiology* (cause); that must be done by diagnostic evalua-

Table 3-2 Some Causes of Symptomatic Localization-Related Epilepsies

Vascular	**Tumors**
• Stroke	• Meningiomas
• Infantile hemiplegia	• Gliomas
• Arteriovenous malformations	• Hamartomas
• Sturge-Weber syndrome	• Metastatic tumors
• Aneurysms (subarachnoid hemorrhage)	
• Venous thrombosis	**Degenerative**
• Hypertensive encephalopathy	• Alzheimer's disease
• Blood dyscrasias (sickle cell anemia)	• Multiple sclerosis
Infectious	**Congenital**
• Abscess	• Heterotopias
• Meningitis and encephalitis	• Cortical dysplasias
• Toxoplasmosis	
• Rubella	**Traumatic**
• Cysticercosis	• Prenatal and perinatal injuries
	• Head injuries
	Cryptogenic
	• No cause identified

tion. The underlying pathology may be diffuse or *multifocal*, such as anoxia (lack of oxygen), physical trauma (head injury), or infections. Other causes are more focal, such a cerebrovascular disease (stroke, arteriovenous malformations, subarachnoid hemorrhage, venous thrombosis), brain tumors (astrocytomas, meningiomas, glioblastomas, metastatic tumors), and mesial temporal sclerosis. Mesial temporal sclerosis may be one of the most surgically treatable of the epilepsies, and will be discussed more fully in Chapter 5.

Despite careful history-taking and the use of improved diagnostic techniques, the cause of epilepsy cannot be determined in many cases. These cases are classified as *cryptogenic* (*crypt* = hidden, *genic* = causative). Consequently, epilepsy of undetermined origin (symptomatic cryptogenic epilepsy) is still the most common syndrome in this category. However, with high-resolution MRI scans, small changes in the organization of gray matter (neurons) are now being recognized in many patients with previously diagnosed cryptogenic epilepsy, allowing the epilepsy to be categorized more specifically.

Epileptic syndromes are often age-specific. Indeed, some syndromes start in childhood, and their natural history is that children outgrow the seizures. Knowing the epileptic syndrome can help predict the future course of the seizures.

GENERALIZED SYNDROMES

The generalized epilepsies are the most common in the pediatric population. *Idiopathic* (genetic) syndromes have been well defined in the last few years, and gene foci have been mapped for some—firmly cementing the concept of a specific, identifiable syndrome.

Juvenile myoclonic epilepsy (JME) has its onset during the teenage years, but persists throughout adulthood and may be lifelong. It consists of a triad of seizures (myoclonic, absence, and generalized tonic-clonic). Myoclonic seizures usually occur in the morning and involve primarily the upper extremities. The most common complaint is clumsiness, or jitters, which is exacerbated by stress and is often initially mistaken for adolescent behavior. Generalized tonic-clonic seizures usually develop in the

35

morning. Absence seizures may be relatively difficult to detect. Not all persons have all three seizure types, but the EEG characteristics—along with the patient's history—are usually diagnostic. It is important to differentiate this syndrome from localization-related epilepsies because treatment is highly specific. Carbamazepine and phenytoin may worsen seizures, while valproate is very effective. A specific gene locus in Chromosome 6p21.2p11 has been proposed for this familial syndrome.

Febrile seizures (febrile convulsions) occur among children from ages 3 months to 5 years who have fever and no evidence of another cause. Today, febrile seizures are not classified as epilepsy but are considered as an age-specific sensitivity of the brain to fever. Usually there are no later consequences. However, many people with *mesial* temporal sclerosis have a history of convulsions in childhood associated with fever, with complex partial seizures beginning in the teenage years and persisting into adulthood.

CASE REPORTS ILLUSTRATING THE USE OF SEIZURE AND EPILEPSY SYNDROME CLASSIFICATION

Case 1

A 36-year-old, right-handed construction worker had been suffering from pounding headaches, often brought on by exertion, for about one year. He also noticed that he did not seem to have the strength and coordination in his left hand that he was accustomed to having. He occasionally found that his left hand would "jerk" for a few seconds. This became progressively worse, but he did not seek medical attention until he had a generalized tonic-clonic seizure at home. He was admitted to the hospital for evaluation and treatment. A CT scan showed a vascular lesion in the right frontal region extending to the motor area. A CT scan with contrast demonstrated this to be an arteriovenous malformation (AVM).

He was initially treated with phenobarbital and phenytoin. Consideration was given to surgery, but it was deemed too risky because of the AVM's large size and its involvement of the motor area. He has been well controlled for the last 12 years and has not had any more generalized tonic-clonic seizures. He continues to have periodic simple partial seizures. He also continues to have intermittent headaches and has had some mild decrease of function in his left hand.

Seizure types: Simple partial seizures with motor symptoms (I.A.1.) and secondarily generalized tonic-clonic seizures (I.C.).

Epileptic syndrome: Localization-relation symptomatic.

Etiology: Arteriovenous malformation.

Prognosis: Lifelong risk for seizures with possible worsening of motor dysfunction and intracerebral hemorrhage from the AVM.

Case 2

A 28-year-old woman was shot in the head (the occipital area) during an airplane hijacking and rendered unconscious. She recovered consciousness many hours later. The bullet had not penetrated her skull. Some months later she began to see "rainbows" lasting from 2 to 5 minutes. She also seemed to experience some loss of vision. These symptoms, which were similar to migrainous phenomena, were not followed by headaches, although she had intermittent neuralgic occipital pain.

A few months later she had a generalized tonic-clonic seizure. EEG revealed occipital spikes. Initial treatment was with phenytoin. This failed to completely control her partial seizures, so carbamazepine was added. The two drugs in combination effectively controlled her seizures. One year later she was admitted to the hospital emergency department with continuous convulsions. Her phenytoin and carbamazepine concentrations were in the therapeutic range. Video EEG showed no epileptiform activity during the seizures. Counseling for post-traumatic stress syndrome was instituted because it was clear that she was suffering from nonepileptic seizures of psychogenic origin. About 2 years after onset, she stopped having simple partial seizures, and the dose of phenytoin was gradually reduced and then eliminated. Her dose of carbamazepine was then reduced to obtain levels of 4–6 mg/L. Over time, her propensity to have seizures decreased as the brain healed. She is now having no seizures and leading an active life with a career and a family. She is a motivational speaker and has written a book on how she overcame the emotional impact of having seizures.

Seizure types: Simple partial seizures with sensory symptoms (I.A.2); secondarily generalized tonic-clonic seizures (I.C.) and nonepileptic seizures.

Epileptic syndrome: Localization-related, symptomatic, and nonepileptic psychogenic.

Etiology: Post-traumatic (for epileptic seizures) and stress (for nonepileptic seizures).

Prognosis: Improvement over time.

Case 3

A 7-year-old girl had a sudden decline in school performance. Her teacher noted frequent episodes of staring and blinking. A physician, suspicious of absence seizures, ordered an EEG. This was normal until she began hyperventilating, which induced an absence seizure with 3-per-second spike-and-wave discharges. She was treated with ethosuximide. Her school performance returned to its normal level. When she was 12 years old, the medication was tapered and then discontinued. EEG was normal both during rest and hyperventilation.

Seizure type: Absence (II.A).

Epileptic syndrome: Childhood absence epilepsy.

Etiology: Idiopathic.

Prognosis: Remission.

REFERENCES

1. Nink-Pflug, J. *Miles to Go Before I Sleep: My Grateful Journey Back from the Hijacking of Egyptair Flight 648*. Center City, MN: Hazelden Foundation, 1996.
2. Commission on Classification and Terminology the International League Against Epilepsy: proposal for the classification of epilepsy and epileptic syndromes. *Epilepsia* 1989;30:389–399.

CHAPTER 4

Treatment of Epilepsy with Drugs

MEDICINES FOR EPILEPSY

B Y FAR THE MOST COMMON treatment for epilepsy is the use of prescription antiepileptic drugs, often abbreviated as AEDs. The AEDs available today have been tested very carefully, and some have been used for many years.

All of the widely used AEDs, except phenobarbital, have been tested in animals before being used in humans. All new drugs are required to be tested first in animals for safety and effectiveness. Only those found to be promising are then tested in human volunteers and then progressively in more and more persons with epilepsy. Often, a substance that has promise in earlier studies is found in human testing to not work well or to have too many side effects, in which case these drugs are not allowed to be used. Each drug approved by the U.S. Food and Drug Administration (FDA) has been tested carefully in hundreds or thousands of persons with epilepsy before being released for marketing.

The obvious ideal is for a new drug to be perfectly 100 percent safe, but this would require much more testing than is practical. At the present time, the FDA requires that an approved drug have a less than a one-in-500 chance of serious side effects. This requires testing in at least 2,000 people. This means, unfortunately, that a new drug still may be responsible for serious side effects in a few people out of thousands, and this may not be discovered until the AED is in wider use. Drugs used today have a very favorable risk-to-reward ratio; this means that the risk from the drug is much smaller than the reward of controlling the seizures. Nevertheless, one must always be aware than any drug for any purpose can cause a rare but serious reaction.

How Do Drugs Work?

As described in Chapter 1, each neuron is an electrochemical cell that can discharge and send a signal to other neurons or cells. Neuron discharging can set off other neurons and cause them to become overexcited. This may result in a seizure. AEDs act by binding to various parts of the neurons to modify their activity and prevent seizures by limiting excitability. Some AEDs work primarily to normalize the firing pattern of neurons that are overexcited, while others block the spread of excessive activity.

The ideal drug should work by blocking abnormal activity without interfering with normal functioning. Many AEDs work at the sodium channel by allowing it to fire at normal rates but by slowing down firing that is too fast. In this way, the spread of overexcited activity is slowed down. AEDs that work at the sodium channel are usually quite effective at blocking the secondarily generalized tonic-clonic seizures in a person with localization-related epilepsy, but they make primary generalized tonic-clonic and myoclonic seizures worse. Other AEDs work at the chloride channel to let more chloride into the neurons, making them more negatively charged and less excitable. These AEDs are particularly useful for primary generalized tonic-clonic seizures but also work to control other types. Some AEDs work primarily at the calcium channel. Other AEDs work by altering the release of the neurotransmitter chemicals from the synapse, and still others work by slowing down the elimination of the neurotransmitters. Most AEDs may work by more than one mechanism, and there are still undiscovered actions. Every available AED has a special mechanism of action that is unique. Fortunately, this gives the physician a large selection of treatments.

Why Do I Need to Take My Medicines Regularly?

Your medicine to control seizures can only work if the right amount is at the place in the brain where it is able to block the start of a seizure or to stop its spread. If medicines are not taken regularly, the amount in the brain can drop to where there is not enough to stop seizures. The major cause of unexpected seizures is missing medicines. The serious and sometimes fatal condition of repeated seizures (*status epilepticus*) can be caused by missing too many doses of medicine (Chapter 11).

How Do Medicines Get into My Body?

The most common way for medicines to get into the body is by swallowing a tablet or capsule. (See Figure 4-1.) Some people have trouble swallowing, so many medicines also are made as a liquid or a chewable tablet. Some capsules have small beads of medicine that can be sprinkled on food. This is especially useful for babies or young children who can eat their medicine with their food.

After swallowing, the medicine goes into the stomach. (See Figure 4-2.) There, the tablets break up into smaller pieces. Capsules, which have a gelatin-like shell, will have the cover digested to release the medicine. Some medicines can leave a burning feeling in the stomach, so they have a type of coating that will not be digested by stomach acids but will break up only after it leaves the stomach and goes into the intestines.

After the medicine breaks up, it must be dissolved in the liquid in the stomach or intestine. The medicines that break up in the stomach can

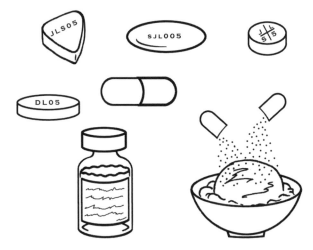

FIGURE 4-1

Antiepileptic drugs come in many forms. Most are tablets of various sizes, shapes, and colors. Others are capsules that can be pulled open so that beads of medicine can be sprinkled on food. Others are liquid.

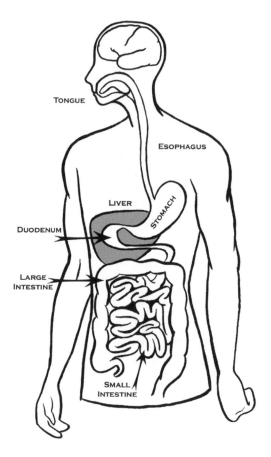

FIGURE 4-2

TONGUE

ESOPHAGUS

LIVER

STOMACH

DUODENUM

LARGE INTESTINE

SMALL INTESTINE

How medicine gets to the brain. After swallowing, medicine goes to the stomach and intestine. There it passes into the blood stream, which takes it to the liver. After the liver processes some of it, the AED goes to the heart and then to the brain.

cross the lining of the stomach into the bloodstream starting only a few minutes after they are swallowed. These medicines often reach their highest amount (maximum concentration, or C_{max}) in 30 to 60 minutes. The time to reach the maximum concentration (T_{max}) is different for each medicine. For medicines that are absorbed into the blood in the intestines, the T_{max} can be as long as 8 to 10 hours.

All medicines that are absorbed in the stomach or intestines (small and large) pass into the portal vein, which goes to the liver. The liver is a large organ that acts like a chemical factory. One of its many jobs is to change (metabolize) things that are not identified as food in order to allow the body to get rid of them. After passing through the liver, medicines then enter the bloodstream to be taken to the heart. The heart pumps the blood containing the medicine to all parts of the body; the brain, kidneys, ovaries, muscle, fat, skin, etc.

Because the brain is so important, about 20% of all of the blood pumped by the heart goes to it. However, because the liver has already metabolized some of the drug, less medicine is now available. For some medicines, the liver metabolizes a lot of it right away (first-pass effect). Medicines that are not swallowed, but are given rectally, absorbed in the mouth, nose, lungs, or skin, or given intravenously or intramuscularly, go directly to the heart and do not have a first-pass effect. For emergency use, medicines can be given intravenously (IV). This shortens the time it takes for the medicine to get to the brain to less than a few seconds and avoids going through the liver first.

After a medicine is in the tissue (brain, muscle, fat, etc.), it slowly re-enters the blood through the veins and is pumped back to the right side of the heart. Some of it goes back to the liver, which metabolizes some more of the drug. The rest goes back to the tissue and some also goes from the tissue back to the blood. This cycle is continuous, and the AED is gradually metabolized by the liver and finally eliminated by the kidney. Some medicines do not get metabolized, but pass from the kidney directly into the urine. In either case, if no medicine is taken to replace the medicine that is being eliminated, the blood level drops over time.

The time it takes for the blood level of a medicine to reach one-half of a previous level is called the half-life $(T_{1/2})$. This time is different for each medicine. Some have a short half-life of 6 to 10 hours, but others have a long half-life of many days. Medicines that have a short half-life need to be taken more often than medicines with a very long half-life. This is why a patient may need to take some medicines many times a day and others only once a day.

As you can see from Figure 4-3, each medicine has its own pattern over time (pharmacokinetic parameter). This determines how the medicines are used. Medicines with a short T_{max} are good for emergency use; those with a long T_{max} are good for oral use. The goal of taking medicines at regular times is to keep the blood level and therefore the brain level in a range that is not too low or too high, as shown in Figure 4-4.

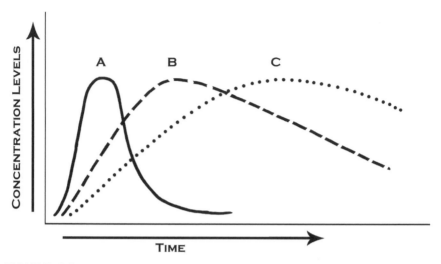

FIGURE 4-3

Drug concentrations over time. Drug A has a short T_{max} and short half-life, and will need to be taken often. Drug C has a long T_{max} and a long half-life and can be taken once a day.

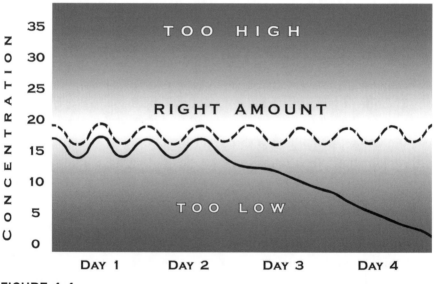

FIGURE 4-4

Measuring drug concentrations in blood. The ideal is to have the right amount, but missing medicines may cause the levels to be too low and result in seizures. Too high and there may be side-effects. The solid line shows what happens if no more medicine is taken after day 2.

A History of the Treatment of Epilepsy

The first effective drug for treatment of epileptic seizures was bromide, introduced in 1857. Before bromide, almost every conceivable potion, diet, and ritual had been used without significant benefit. Although effective for controlling seizures, bromide's side effects are considerable and include sedation, depression, skin rashes, and gastro-intestinal distress. For more than 60 years, bromide was the only effective substance known for the treatment of epilepsy.

Because sedation was a prominent side effect of bromide, it was considered to be essential for its anticonvulsant effect. Based on this concept, phenobarbital was introduced for the treatment of epilepsy in 1912. For the next 25 years, epilepsy was treated with drugs associated with slowing of mentation (mental activity) and, in retrospect, the belief that persons with epilepsy were mentally subnormal may have been a result of the treatment rather than the disorder.

Today, it is difficult to imagine that substances to treat illnesses could be given to humans before being thoroughly tested in animals for safety and efficacy, but this had been the case for millennia. The FDA was authorized by Congress in the early 1930s with a mandate to approve only medicines that had been tested for safety. Because of a law exempting them, natural products do not have to be tested for safety, although many of them have been found to be dangerous.

Phenytoin was the first drug to be extensively tested in animals. It was found to lack sedative effects. From 1946 to 1978, other substances were approved for marketing in the United States. Some have been withdrawn because of toxicity, and many of the others have been found to have only limited use. From 1961 through 1973, no major new drugs for epilepsy were marketed in the United States, although carbamazepine, valproate, and other agents were being used in other countries. Carbamazepine was approved for marketing in the United States in 1974. Valproate was approved in 1978. In the interim, there were no new major drugs approved for the treatment of epilepsy until 1993—a significant lapse of 15 years.

Starting in the late 1970s, there was renewed interest in developing new drugs for epilepsy treatment in the United States. The Epilepsy

Branch of the National Institutes of Health began a comprehensive system for screening promising compounds in animal models of epilepsy. More than 30,000 compounds have been screened, and from these a few were promising enough to warrant testing in humans. During the past decade, more than 21 compounds have been tested in humans in the United States, but not all have made it to use. The FDA approved felbamate and gabapentin in 1993, lamotrigine in 1994, topiramate and fosphenytoin in 1996, tiagabine in 1997, levetiracetam in 1999, and oxcarbazepine and zonisamide in 2000 and pregabalin in 2005. Some other new drugs are now in clinical trails in the United States. (See Table 4-1.)

In addition to AEDs, many other substances can alter brain activity. Some can influence the brain to become more excitable. These include some prescription drugs and "natural" products such as ephedra, *ma huang*, bitter orange, and excessive caffeine. These may cause seizures by disturbing the normal balance between the excitatory and inhibitory chemicals in the brain, even when AEDs are being used.

SIDE EFFECTS

Drugs, when absorbed, travel to all parts of the body and brain, so they can have a number of effects that are not related to their intended purpose. Although some of these unintended effects may lead to other uses

Table 4-1 Most Common Antiepileptic Drugs Marketed in the United States

Year Introduced	Name	Year Introduced	Name
1912	Phenobarbital	1993	Felbamate
1938	Phenytoin		Gabapentin
1954	Primidone	1994	Lamotrigine
1960	Ethosuximide	1996	Topiramate
1968	Diazepam	1997	Tiagabine
1974	Carbamazepine	1999	Levetiracetam
1975	Clonazepam	2000	Oxcarbazepine
1978	Valproate		Zonisamide
		2005	Pregabalin

(e.g., gabapentin for pain, valproate for depression), these are termed adverse effects. Adverse effects can be related to high levels or they can happen even at small doses (idiosyncratic or allergic), and they may limit the usefulness of a drug. All drugs to treat epilepsy work in the brain, and many of the unintended effects relate to normal functioning of the brain.

There is a direct relation between the level of a drug and its effects. If the level is too low, it is considered to be subtherapeutic. The level at which a drug works as intended but does not cause adverse effects is called the therapeutic range, and the level above this is called the toxic range. (Figure 4-4). Many drugs used for epilepsy have therapeutic ranges available. However, these ranges are based on how groups of people have reacted to the drug and should not be used as absolute values to treat individuals.

For example, the most common therapeutic range for phenytoin is given as 10 to 20 mg/L. However, some persons with hard-to-control seizures have the best results with levels higher than 20 mg/L. Some persons are very sensitive to side effects and may have trouble at levels below 20 mg/L. The best way to use blood levels is to measure them when the person is doing well and use that as the target range for that individual. When a seizure then occurs, blood levels should be measured; often, the level is found to be much lower than that person's range. This means the seizure was probably caused by missed medication. The goal is for each person to have his or her own individual therapeutic range identified.

Because the brain controls mood, behavior, thinking, and sleep, common side effects of drugs used to treat epilepsy include depression, aggressive behavior, slow thinking, and sleepiness. The goal of treatment is to control seizures without causing side effects—"no seizures/no side effects." This is often possible, but it may be tricky. Not everyone experiences the same side effects from each medicine. The best approach is for the physician to choose a group of medicines that are effective for the type of epilepsy. The potential for side effects should be reviewed, and those drugs that may have negative effects should be avoided. (For example, women who wish to have children should avoid medicines that may cause birth defects.) Then, a dose to get to the usual effective range should be chosen.

Side effects can be confusing. This is especially true for drugs used to treat seizures because many of their side effects involve things many people feel normally, such as being tired, sleepy, having trouble concentrating, feeling depressed, or otherwise not feeling well. Most of these side effects depend on how much of the drug is in the body, and changing the dose may help in reducing the side effects. Some drugs have more side effects than others, and some people are sensitive to one drug but may not be sensitive to another. For that reason, it is important to discuss one's comfort level with the physician. In some cases, to get complete seizure control, very high doses of medicine are needed and having side effects constantly may be worse than having an occasional seizure. A balance of the fewest seizures and tolerable side effects that is best for each person must be reached.

To help better understand side effects, the following discussion will be organized by organ systems:

SIDE EFFECTS INVOLVING THE BRAIN

Because the brain controls our thinking processes, emotions, motor activities, and senses, AEDs can affect these. Almost everyone who takes AEDs may experience side effects in some of these areas. These are usually most troublesome at the beginning of treatment and may lessen and disappear with time. Some medicines need to be started with smaller doses, which are gradually increased over a few weeks, while others can be started at effective doses at the beginning. Most of these side effects are not dangerous, although they can be troublesome.

The most common side effects are sleepiness, fatigue, lack of energy, slowed thinking, an inability to concentrate, and physical weakness. Mood change for the worse (irritability, crankiness, depression, aggressiveness) or mood change for the better (less anxiety, less depression) can also occur. Most of the drugs used to treat epilepsy are also used to treat other conditions, so sometimes one drug can be chosen to treat two conditions. For example, valproate is also indicated for manic-depressive illness, and a physician may choose it over other AEDs if a person has both disorders.

Most of the AEDs when present at high levels will cause trouble with balance (ataxia) and coordination. These effects are similar to effects from alchohol intoxication, and physicians often use "the drunk test" (walking in a straight line) to examine a person in the clinic for these effects. Another common side effect is nystagmus (jerky vision). These effects can usually be eliminated by decreasing the dose or using a different AED. Tremor is also a common side effect of many of the AEDs (Figure 4-4).

SIDE EFFECTS AFFECTING THE SKIN

Most medicines can cause skin rashes. AEDs are not unusual in this regard. For some AEDs, as many as 4–6 persons out of 100 (4–6%) may experience an allergic rash, whereas for other AEDs, allergic rashes are very rare. Most skin rashes from AEDs are not related to the dose or level (they are idiosyncratic) and appear within one to two weeks after starting the drug. It is a good idea to check the skin before starting a medicine because normally many people have slight rashes or acne (pimples). Checking the skin carefully before starting treatment with AEDs will help prevent unnecessary concern over rashes that may not have been noticed before the treatment began.

Drug rashes usually appear first on the back and chest, and the first symptom is itching. The rashes appear as reddened areas the size of a small pea but may become larger. Skin of the arms and legs may also be affected without affecting the palms of the hands or the soles of the feet. The face is usually less involved. Fever, if present, is usually not severe. The rash usually worsens over a 24–48 hour period. If a rash develops, the AED should be stopped and a visit to the physician or medical facility should be made to determine if the rash is from the AED and, if so, if a different AED should be started. If the rash was from the AED, it should be listed as an allergic reaction. Most rashes happen 1 to 2 weeks after starting the AED. Rashes that start months after starting an AED are usually not caused by the drug. Nevertheless, they should be evaluated.

Like other drugs, AEDs can sometimes be associated with very serious and even fatal skin reactions (e.g., Stevens–Johnson syndrome).

This may happen during the first few weeks or sometimes much later. This often involves the palms of the hands and soles of the feet and may affect the linings of the mouth. Hospitalization is usually necessary in this case, and the sooner the drug is stopped, the better the outcome. It may be fatal.

SIDE EFFECTS INVOLVING THE LIVER

Many commonly used medicines, such as acetaminophen, can cause liver damage. Some AEDs can do so as well. The risk of liver failure may be as high as 1 out of 200 children under the age of two from valproate, or it can be extremely rare. In most cases, liver damage starts a few weeks or months after starting a drug, but in a few cases it may be years later. Liver damage can often be detected by blood tests. One should have a liver test before starting an AED and then again a few months later. If these tests are normal, later routine tests for most AEDs are not useful and add to the cost of care. However, if one develops unusual nausea, loss of appetite, jaundice (skin or whites of eyes turning yellow), severe tiredness or other unusual symptoms, a liver test should be done immediately.

SIDE EFFECTS INVOLVING THE BLOOD SYSTEM

The blood contains white blood cells (WBC) that fight infections, red blood cells (RBC) that carry oxygen, and platelets that cause the blood to clot. These are manufactured by the bone marrow. Some drugs can damage the bone marrow, causing some or all of the blood cells to decrease or vanish. A small decrease in the WBC count may occur with some AEDs, but this may not be serious and the AED may not have to be stopped. A complete blood count (CBC) should be obtained before trying any AED and repeated in 3–6 months. For most AEDs, it is then not necessary to repeat the CBC routinely, but should be done as soon as possible if signs develop.

The most common adverse side effect of AEDs for the blood system are new signs of bleeding, excessive bleeding during menstrual periods, small cuts that are not healing, signs of a petechial rash (small, pinpoint spots of red on the skin), or blood in the urine. If these occur, a CBC should be done immediately.

The most severe type of reaction of the bone marrow is called aplastic anemia. It may normally occur with no known cause in 2–4 persons in a million. However, with felbamate it may happen in 1 in 5,000 people. For some of the other AEDs, aplastic anemia may occur in 1 in 200,000.

SPECIFIC ANTI-EPILEPTIC DRUGS

Until 10 years ago, the choice of medicines was limited to three or four, with only a few mechanisms of action, but in the last decade a number of new drugs have become available. This is an astonishing improvement in treatment, especially in view of the fact that there were no new drugs for epilepsy from 1978 to 1993. Because each drug is unique in its profile of effectiveness and side effects, the possibility of matching up a drug with each individual for the best outcome is now greater than ever before. The cost of developing drugs and concern about high prices of drugs make it unlikely that we will have another decade during which so many new drugs for epilepsy will be developed.

This section will describe the most widely used drugs to treat epilepsy in alphabetical order using their generic names. Most of the newer drugs do not yet have generics available. Soon, however, many will have generics, and the brands may develop different formulations, so interested persons should check with their pharmacist about availability.

CARBAMAZEPINE

Action and Uses

Carbamazepine is effective for simple (IA) and complex partial seizures (IB) and secondarily (IC) (Table 2-1) generalized tonic-clonic seizures. It is not effective for absence, myoclonic, or atonic seizures and may cause some generalized tonic-clonic seizures to worsen.

Available Formations

Tablets:

    Generic: tablets 200 mg; chewable 100 mg

    Brand: Tegretol®: 200 mg; chewable 100 mg

Extended Release:

    Generic: none

    Brand: Carbatrol®: 100, 200, 300 mg.

             Tegretol® XR: tablets 100, 200, 400 mg.

Suspension

    100 mg per 5 ml

Intravenous

    None available (being developed)

Absorption

Time to peak plasma concentrations (T_{max}) is 4 to 12 hours after use of solid dosage forms. Because of its short half-life and rapid absorption rate, wide variations may occur between peak and trough levels. To overcome this, extended release forms, Tegretol® XR and Carbatrol®, were developed. These have the advantage of providing steadier levels, leading to fewer side effects as peak concentrations are avoided. Better seizure control is also possible because low levels before the next dose are avoided. With monotherapy (the use of one drug), the usual effective plasma concentration is 4 to 12 mg/L, but higher concentrations may be required in some patients to control seizures. With concomitant use of other AEDs, lower concentrations may be associated with toxicity.

Metabolism

Carbamazepine is metabolized in the liver to its 10,11-epoxide. This compound has both anticonvulsant and toxic effects. Carbamazepine induces its own metabolism. As a result, the usual initial half-life of 18 to 35 hours is reduced considerably after 3 or 4 weeks of use. Use of phenytoin or phenobarbital with carbamazepine speeds up its metabolism so higher doses may be required when used in combination.

Dosage and Administration

Children 6–12 years, 100 mg twice daily on the first day. The amount can be increased by 100 mg daily at appropriate intervals (usually 1–2 weeks) and given in three or four divided doses until the desired response is obtained. The usual daily maintenance dose is 400–800 mg (15 to 30 mg/kg); the frequency of administration must be individualized. For children 4–6 years, 10–20 mg/kg in two or three divided doses is warranted, increased by up to 100 mg daily at weekly intervals, as needed and tolerated. The usual maintenance dose is 250–350 mg a day (usual maximum dose, 400 mg). For children under 4 years, an initial dose of 20–60 mg is recommended.

For adults and adolescents, initially 400 mg should be divided into two doses on the first day, increased by 200 mg daily at appropriate intervals (usually 1–2 weeks) and administered in three or four divided doses to minimize the peak and trough effects. Extended release formulations may be given only twice a day—morning and night. The usual daily maintenance dose is 600 mg to 1.2 g in monotherapy, but may be as high as 2.0 g in combination therapy. Elderly patients metabolize carbamazepine more slowly and therefore will need lower doses.

Side Effects

Many people have few or no side effects. The most common side effects that occur during early treatment with carbamazepine are drowsiness, dizziness, lightheadedness, diplopia (seeing double), ataxia (trouble with balance), nausea, and vomiting. These usually either decrease or disappear within a week or after a reduction in dose. Much rarer and more serious side effects involve the skin, bone marrow, and liver.

Almost 2 to 4 persons in a hundred will have a skin rash involving the back and chest about 2 weeks after starting carbamazepine. This usually is not dangerous, but the drug should be stopped and the patient should notify his or her physician. About one person in 100,000 using carbamazepine may develop a very serious and possibly fatal skin reaction (Stevens–Johnson syndrome).

Gastrointestinal reactions include gastric distress and abdominal pain, diarrhea, constipation, and anorexia. Dryness of the mouth and soreness of the tongue also can occur.

A small decrease in the white blood count occurs in approximately 10% of patients treated with carbamazepine, but discontinuance of the drug usually is not required. Other reactions involving the blood (aplastic anemia) are rare, but they may be fatal. Because their onset maybe gradual and is reversible when the drug is discontinued, patients should notify their physician promptly if fever, easy bruising, petechial spots, or other unusual signs appear.

Carbamazepine may cause low sodium levels in the serum because of its effect on the action on a hormone that regulates water balance (antidiuretic hormone). This happens in fewer than 5 persons in 100, but is most likely to happen to those who drink abnormal amounts of liquid, are taking medicines to get rid of water (diuretics) or are older (over 50).

Cardiovascular, genitourinary, metabolic, hepatic, and other reactions have been reported rarely. These include aggravation of hypertension or ischemic heart disease, arrhythmias, hypotension, syncope, edema, congestive heart failure, recurrence of thrombophlebitis, urinary frequency, acute urinary retention, albuminuria, glycosuria, elevated blood urea nitrogen levels, microscopic deposits in the urine, impotence, jaundice, myalgia (muscle pain) and arthralgia, leg cramps, and conjunctivitis.

Drug Interactions

Approximately 75% of carbamazepine is bound to plasma albumin, but this is not clinically significant. As a result of enzyme induction, carbamazepine increases the hepatic metabolism of many drugs (Table 4-2). Valproate has a variable effect on carbamazepine steady-state concentrations and decreases carbamazepine epoxide metabolism, which may have therapeutic or toxic significance. Carbamazepine concentrations are markedly increased by erythromycin (an antibiotic) and propoxyphene hydrochloride (a painkiller, brand name Darvon). Other drugs may have lesser effects. Carbamazepine also may reduce

Table 4-2 Clinically Significant Drug Interactions

Drug and Isoenzyme	Levels increased by	Levels decreased by	Effect on other drugs	
			Increases	Decreases
Carbamazepine	Erythromycin	Phenobarbital		Clonazepam
CYP 3A4/5 sub+ind	Clarithromycin	Phenytoin		Ethosuximide
CYP 2D6 ind	Isoniaid			Primidone
CYP 2C9 ind	Propoxyphene			Valproate
CYP 1A2 ind	Troleandomycin			Topiramate
CYP 2C19 ind	Cimetidine			Phenytoin
	Danazol			Phenobarbital
	Diltiazem			Oral contraceptives
	Verapamil			Disopyramide
	Fluoxetine			Rifampin
	Sertraline			Ketoconazole
	Fluvoxamine			Meperidine
	Indinavir			Warfarin
	Grapefruit juice			
				Tacrolimus
				Protease inhibitors
				Trazodone
				Quinidine
Ethosuximide		Carbamazepine		
CYP 3A4 sub		Phenobarbital		
		Phenytoin		
		Primidone		

(continued on next page)

Table 4-2 Clinically Significant Drug Interactions (continued)

Drug and Isoenzyme	Levels increased by	Levels decreased by	Effect on other drugs	
			Increases	**Decreases**
Felbamate CYP 2C19 blk		Phenytoin Phenobarbital Carbamazepine	Phenytoin Valproate Carbamazepine epoxide	Carbamazepine
Gabapentin No hepatic metabolism				
Lamotrigine	Valproate	Phenytoin Carbamazepine		
Levetiracetam No significant hepatic metabolism				
Oxcarbazepine CYP 3A4, 5-7 ind CYP 2C19 blk		Phenytoin Carbamazepine Phenobarbital	Phenytoin	Clonazepam Ethosuximide Primidone Valproate Topiramate Phenytoin Phenobarbital Oral contraceptives Disopyramide Rifampin Ketoconazole Meperidine Warfarin Tacrolimus

Table 4-2 Clinically Significant Drug Interactions (continued)

Drug and Isoenzyme	Levels increased by	Levels decreased by	Effect on other drugs	
			Increases	Decreases
				Protease inhibitors
				Trazodone
				Quinidine
Phenobarbital/Primidone		Phenytoin		Topiramate
CYP 1A2, 2B6, 2C8-10,		Carbamazepine		Carbamazepine
3A4, 3A5-7 ind				Phenobarbital
				Primidone
				Valproate
				Oral contraceptives
				Disopyramide
				Quinidine
				Ketoconazole
				Itraconazole
				Etoposide
				Corticosteroids
				Warfarin
				Trazodone
				Cyclosporine
				Tacrolimus
				Protease inhibitors
				Methadone
				Propafenone
				Theophylline

(continued on next page)

Table 4-2 Clinically Significant Drug Interactions (continued)

Drug and Isoenzyme	Levels increased by	Levels decreased by	Increases	Decreases
Phenytoin CYP 2C9, 2C19 sub+ind CYP 3A4/5 ind CYP 2D6 ind CYP 2A2 ind	Topiramate Chloramphenicol Cimetidine Dicumarol Disulfiram Isoniazid Phenylbutazone Sulfonamides Trimethoprim Amiodarone Allopurinol Chlorpheniramine Fluoxetine Fluvoxamine Ranitidine Omeprazole Fluconazole	Carbamazepine Phenobarbital Valproate Diazoxide Antineoplastics Loxepine Rifampin		Topiramate Carbamazepine Phenobarbital Primidone Valproate Oral contraceptives Disopyramide Quinidine Ketoconazole Itraconazole Etoposide Corticosteroids Warfarin Trazodone Cyclosporine Tacrolimus Protease inhibitors Methadone Propafenone Theophylline
Pregabaline No hepatic metabolism				

(continued on next page)

Table 4-2 Clinically Significant Drug Interactions (continued)

Drug and Isoenzyme	Levels increased by	Levels decreased by	Effect on other drugs	
			Increases	Decreases
Tiagabine		Phenytoin Carbamazepine Phenobarbital		
Topiramate CYP 3A sub		Phenytoin Carbamazepine	Phenytoin	
Valproate 2C9 blk		Carbamazepine Phenobarbital Primidone Phenytoin Salicyclates	Lamotrigine Phenobarbital Carbamazepine Carbamazepine epoxide	Phenytoin Ehtosuximide
Zonisamide CYP 2C19 sub CYP 2D6 sub CYP 3A4 sub		Carbamazepine Phenytoin Phenobarbital		

Note: Isoenzymes are the specific subunits of the liver that metabolize the listed AEDs. New information about drug interactions is being developed constantly. Isoenzymes are under genetic control and in the future persons can be tested to find out if they have a problem before the medicine is used.

the plasma concentration and therapeutic response to corticosteroids or thyroid hormones. The combination of carbamazepine and lithium may increase the risk of neurotoxicity.

CLONAZEPAM

Action and Uses

Clonazepam (Klonopin®) is sometimes used alone or in combination with other drugs to control myoclonic or atonic seizures and photosensitive epilepsy. In patients with juvenile myoclonic epilepsy, clonazepam may help control myoclonic jerks.

Available Formations

Tablets
    Generic: Tablets 0.5,1, and 2 mg
    Brand: Klonopin®: tablets 0.5, 1, and 2 mg

Absorption

Peak plasma concentrations occur 1–4 hours after oral administration. It is almost completely biotransformed to inactive metabolites. The reported half-life ranges are similar for adults (19–50 hours) and children (22–33 hours).

Dosage and Administration

Oral
    Adults: initially 1.5 mg daily in three divided doses, increased by 0.5 to 1 mg every third day until seizures are adequately controlled or until adverse effects occur.
    Children: Doses of 0.5 mg should be used initially.
    Doses for the elderly have not been well established.

Side-Effects

The most common adverse effects of clonazepam involve the central nervous system. Approximately one-half of patients experience some drowsiness, about one-third ataxia, and up to one-quarter personality changes. The sedation may be minimized by initiating therapy with a small dose and increasing the amount gradually.

DIAZEPAM

Actions and Uses

Diazepam preparations are used for emergency treatment of seizures, such as clusters, acute repetitive seizures and status epilepticus. Maintenance therapy with oral diazepam is not useful in treating epilepsy.

Formations Useful for Emergency Treatment of Seizures

Solutions
> Generic: Solution 5 mg/mL in 1-mL, 2-mL, and 10-mL containers.
> Brand: Valium®: Solution 5 mg/mL in 2-mL and 10-mL containers.

Rectal Gel
> Rectal Diastat®: Rectal delivery system, adjustable from 2.5 mg to 10 mg for children, and 10 mg to 20 mg for adults.

Absorption

Liquid oral forms (solutions) are useful for a person who is developing seizures. Giving oral diazepam into the cheek pouch in the mouth may often prevent the need to call 911. Because it goes directly into the blood going to the heart, it does not go to the liver first and works better than a pill. Diazepam's onset of action is almost immediate after intravenous administration. The rectal solution reaches peak concentrations in 5 minutes.

Side Effects

Diazepam may make a person tired or sleepy, but in some children it may have the opposite effect and cause hyperactive behavior.

ETHOSUXIMIDE

Actions and Uses

Ethosuximide (Zarontin®) works mostly for absence seizures unaccompanied by other types of seizures.

Available Formations

Capsules
    Generic: 250 mg
    Brand: Zarontin®: 250 mg
Syrup
    Generic: 250 mg/5ml
    Brand: Zarontin®; 250 mg/5ml

Absorption

Ethosuximide is well absorbed orally, and the T_{max} is 1–4 hours. It is minimally bound to plasma protein and eliminated mostly by liver metabolism. The half-life is averages 52–56 hours in adults and 32–41 hours in children. Control of absence seizures usually is achieved with plasma concentrations of 40–100 mg/L.

Dosage and Administration

Oral
    Adults and children over 6 years of age: Initially 500 mg daily, increased if necessary by 250 mg every 4–7 days until seizures are controlled or until untoward effects develop. The daily maintenance dose is usually 15–40 mg/kg.

Children 3 to 6 years of age: Initially 250 mg daily with incremental increases in dosage, as for older patients. The daily maintenance dose is usually 15–40 mg/kg.

Side Effects

The most common adverse reactions to ethosuximide are gastrointestinal disturbances (e.g., nausea, vomiting).

Drug Interactions

Ethosuximide does not have any significant known drug interactions.

FELBAMATE (FELBATOL®)

Action and Uses

In July 1993, the FDA granted approval of felbamate for both add-on therapy and as monotherapy in adults with partial seizures with or without generalization, and in children with partial and generalized seizures associated with the LennoxGastaut syndrome. However, a strong warning was added in September 1994 because of reports of aplastic anemia and hepatitis. Felbamate should be reserved for those patients for whom there is no other effective alternative treatment.

Available Formations

Felbamate: Felbatol® (MedPointe) tablets, 400 mg, 600 mg; oral suspension 600 mg/5mL.

Absorption

The elimination half-life of felbamate is approximately 15–20 hours. Its pharmacokinetics appear to be linear. Time to maximum concentration occurs 1–4 hours after a dose is administered. Plasma protein binding is not clinically significant.

Doses and Administration

In adults, doses during clinical trials have ranged from 1800 to 4800 mg/day. In children, doses of 15 to 45 mg/kg have been used. With monotherapy, larger doses are tolerated.

Side Effects

Side effects include insomnia, weight loss, nausea, decreased appetite, dizziness, fatigue, ataxia, and lethargy. There were substantially higher rates of side effects in people receiving other antiepileptic medications, and conversion to monotherapy often reduced side effects. Although its use has been limited, no fatalities have been reported with Felbatol since 1994.

Drug Interactions

Felbamate has significant interactions with phenytoin, carbamazepine, and valproate. The concentrations of phenytoin and valproate increase with felbamate. Therefore, when felbamate is initiated, the doses of these other agents should be decreased by 20% to 40% or more. On the other hand, carbamazepine concentrations decrease by about 20% when felbamate is added to therapy. The concentrations of felbamate are lowered by the concomitant use of other antiepileptic drugs, especially those that induce hepatic enzymes.

GABAPENTIN

Action and Uses

The FDA approved gabapentin for use in adults as an add-on therapy for partial and secondarily generalized seizures. Its major difference from other antiepileptic medications is its lack of interactions with other drugs. Since its introduction for use in epilepsy, gabapentin has been shown to be effective in certain chronic pain syndromes. In clinical practice, blood levels of 2–20 mg/L have been found to be effective.

Available Formations

Gelatin capsules and tablets
 Generic: Capsules, 100, 300, 400 mg, and tablets 600 and 800 mg.
 Brand: Neurontin®: capsules, 100, 300, 400 mg, and tablets 600 and 800 mg.
Oral Solution
 250 mg/5ml

Absorption

The oral bioavailability of gabapentin is approximately 60% in humans. The time to maximum concentration is 2–4 hours after a dose is taken. Gabapentin does not bind to human plasma proteins. The renal clearance of gabapentin equals the total clearance in normal volunteers and is 120–130 mL/min. No metabolite has been detected in human beings. After single doses, a linear correlation has been demonstrated between dose and the 2-hour plasma concentration in patients on gabapentin monotherapy.

Doses and Administration

The initial dose of gabapentin in adults is 900 mg/day in divided doses. It can be rapidly titrated, 300 mg on day one, 300 mg t.i.d. day two, and then 300 mg t.i.d. Usual doses for epilepsy are 1800 to 3600 mg/day but doses as high as 6000 mg/day have been well tolerated in adults.

Side Effects

The most common side effects from gabapentin are mild fatigue and dizziness. Other side effects have been nystagmus, hypotension, diarrhea, muscle weakness, dry mouth, sleep disturbances, slurred speech, decreased alertness, tremor, rash, and nausea. There have been no changes in the hematologic and biochemical parameters.

 Gabapentin in very large doses appears to have little toxicity; one patient took 48 g in an attempted suicide. Even though blood levels were initially over 60 mg/L, clearance was rapid and she experienced minimal symptoms.

Drug Interactions

Because of its lack of interaction with other drugs, it is especially useful in patients who are receiving many other medications, such as the elderly.

LAMOTRIGINE

Action and Uses

Clinical studies have demonstrated lamotrigine to be effective in adults with partial and generalized seizures. It was approved for use in December 1994 for adults with complex partial seizures and secondarily generalized seizures.

Available Formations

Tablets
    Generic: Various doses
    Brand: Lamictal® 25, 100, 150, 200 mg; and 2, 5, 25, mg chewable tablets

Absorption and Metabolism

Lamotrigine is rapidly absorbed after oral dosing and is extensively metabolized and excreted predominantly as a glucuronide. In normal volunteers, the mean terminal elimination half-life is 24 hours. Patients receiving either phenytoin or carbamazepine were found to have a shorter half-life, 15 hours (range 7.8 to 33 hours). In patients receiving valproate, the lamotrigine half-life was 59 hours (range 30 to 89 hours). In clinical practice, effective serum concentrations of lamotrigine vary from 2 to 20 mg/L.

Doses and Administration

Doses of 75–600 mg/day have been used in studies of adults with epilepsy, but doses up to 1600 mg may be needed with polytherapy. The initial doses of lamotrigine must be adjusted to concomitant medications. If the patient is on enzyme-inducing antiepileptic drugs but not valproate, the dose should be 50 mg/day for 2 weeks, then 100 mg for the next two weeks, and then the dose can be increased by 100 mg each week to a dose of 300 to 500 mg/day. If the patient is on valproate, the initial dose should be 25 mg every other day for two weeks, then 25 mg/day for the next two weeks, then increased by 25 to 50 mg every week or two to a dose of 100 to 150 mg/day.

Side Effects

The most frequently reported side effects of lamotrigine have been diplopia, drowsiness, ataxia, and headache. A higher incidence of skin rash has been observed in patients receiving concomitant valproic acid. In children, a high rate of serious skin rashes, including Stevens–Johnson syndrome, has occurred. In March 1997, the manufacturer added a warning that the rate of serious rash may occur in 1:50 to 1:100 children. Slow titration appears to lessen the incidence of skin rashes. Clinical experience has shown that serum concentrations between 2.0 and 20.0 mg/L have been effective and tolerated.

Drug Interactions

Lamotrigine does not appear to affect the concentrations of other antiepileptic drugs. However, other drugs affect lamotrigine. Valproate causes a marked prolongation of lamotrigine half-life, to almost double or triple its half-life when used alone. Phenytoin and carbamazepine significantly shorten lamotrigine's half-life. Hormonal contraceptives and pregnancy decrease lamotrigine levels substantially.

LEVETIRACETAM

Actions and Uses

Levetiracetam is indicated for use as adjunctive treatment of partial onset seizures in adults with epilepsy. Its precise mechanism of action is unknown, but it is found in high concentrations in synaptic vesicles and presumed to regulate release of neurostransmitters.

Available Formations

Tablets
    Generic: None
    Brand: Keppra® 250 mg, 500 mg, 750 mg.
Oral Suspension
    100 mg/ml
Intravenous
    100 mg/ml

Absorption and Elimination

Levetiracetam is rapidly absorbed (T_{max} 1 hour after administration) and its oral bioavailability is close to 100%. It is very water soluble, and its volume of distribution similar to that of intracellular and extracellular water. Protein binding is less than 10%. Levetiracetam is not metabolized by the liver and is excreted unchanged in the urine. Its plasma half-life in adults is 6 to 8 hours, but its antiseizure activity is longer.

Doses and Administration

Initial adult doses of levetiracetam at 500 mg b.i.d. Clinical studies have shown 1000 mg/day to be effective. Doses may be increased in increments of 1000 mg/day. The usual dose in adults is 2500 mg/day but higher doses may be needed. Pediatric doses appear to be in the range of 20 to 40 mg/kg/day. In elderly patients and others with decreased renal function, doses need to be reduced.

Side Effects

In placebo-controlled studies, dizziness, somnolence, depression, and changes in behavior were the most commonly reported side effects. The psychiatric reactions, which happen in about 6% of treated patients, stop when levetiracetam is discontinued. No serious idiosyncratic adverse events have been noted.

Drug Interactions

The lack of drug interactions make this a useful AED for patients receiving chemotherapy and elderly receiving many other medicines.

OXCARBAZEPINE

Actions and Uses

Oxcarbazepine has been approved for monotherapy and as adjunctive treatment in partial seizures in adults and children ages 4 to 16.

Available Formations

Tablets
 Generic: None
 Brand: Trileptal® (Novartis) 150, 300, 600 mg;
Suspension
 Brand: Trileptal® (Novartis) 300 mg/5mL

Absorption

Oxcarbazepine is inactive but is metabolized into 10-mono-hydroxy-oxcarbazepine (MHD). Oxcarbazepine is completely absorbed with an average T_{max} of 4.5 hours. It then has a plasma half-life of approximately 2 hours, while MHD has a half-life of approximately 9 hours. Approximately 70% of oxcarbazepine is converted to MHD, the rest to inactive metabolites. Approximately 40% is protein bound.

Dosage and Administration

As monotherapy, treatment with oxcarbazepine should be initiated with a dose of 300 mg b.i.d. in adults, and increased by 300 mg every third day to a dose of 1200 mg/day. As adjunctive therapy, treatment can be initiated at 300 mg b.i.d. and increased as needed. To convert to monotherapy, other AEDs can then be decreased over 3 to 6 weeks, or longer, as clinically indicated. In general, 300 mg of oxcarbazepine is equivalent to 200 mg of carbamazepine.

For children, initial doses should be 8–10 mg/kg/day b.i.d. Doses can be increased to 20–40 mg/kg/day. Children under 8 years of age may need doses 30%–40% greater.

Side Effects

Like carbamazepine, oxcarbazepine may be associated with hyponatremia. In placebo-controlled studies, 38 of 1,524 (2.5%) patients treated with oxcarbazepine had serum sodium concentrations of less than 125 mmol/L (normal 135 to 142 mmol/L) compared to none treated with placebo. In addition, 25%–30% of patients who had a hypersensitivity reaction (skin rash) to carbamazepine developed a similar reaction to oxcarbazepine. Most common side effects are related to the central nervous system and include dizziness, somnolence, diplopia, fatigue, and ataxia.

Drug Interactions

Oxcarbazepine can inhibit CYP 2C10 and induce CYP 3A4/5. Thus, oxcarbazepine may increase phenytoin concentrations (metabolized by CYP 2C19) by as much as 40%. By inducing CYP 3A, hormonal contraceptives may be rendered less effective.

Phenobarbital And Primidone

Actions and Uses

Phenobarbital (phenobarbital sodium), a long-acting barbiturate, is effective in generalized tonic-clonic and simple partial seizures. Phenobarbital frequently is used to treat neonatal seizures. However, because of increasing concern about adverse neuropsychologic reactions to sedative/hypnotic antiepileptic drugs, many clinicians prefer less sedating drugs.

Primidone is active by itself, but its major antiseizure activity and adverse effects arise from being metabolized (converted by the liver) to phenobarbital.

Available Formations

Tablets
   Generic: Phenobarbital 8, 15, 30, 60, and 100 mg;.
   Generic: Primidone 250 mg.
   Brand: Mysoline® 50 and 250 mg.
Suspension
   Generic: Phenobarbital solution 15 and 20 mg/mL;
   Brand: Mysoline® suspension 250 mg/5 mL

Absorption

Phenobarbital is almost completely absorbed orally. It has a T_{max} of 1–6 hours. The average plasma half-life is 3 days in children and 4 days in adults; consequently, 3 or more weeks may be required to attain steady-state plasma concentrations. Plasma concentrations of 15–40 mg/L are usually optimal for the control of epilepsy.

Dosage and Administration

   Phenobarbital: Oral administration. Adults, 120–250 mg; children, 2–3 mg/kg/day.

Primidone: Oral administration. Adults and older children, initially 125 mg at bedtime for 3 days, with the dose increased by 125 mg every 3 days until a maintenance dose of 250 mg three times a day is established on the 10th day.

Side Effects

Phenobarbital and primidone are associated with significant behavioral and cognitive effects. Drowsiness is the most common adverse reaction, although tolerance usually develops, and a significant percentage of patients continue to experience sedation. Furthermore, phenobarbital may affect memory, perceptual motor performance, and tasks requiring sustained performance.

Phenobarbital and primidone can provoke irritability and exacerbate existing behavioral problems, particularly hyperactivity. A substantial number of adults who take phenobarbital develop depression.

Drug Interactions

Phenobarbital both induces hepatic enzymes and competitively inhibits drug biotransformation. Thus, mutual enzyme induction or inhibition in patients treated with phenobarbital and phenytoin may result in an increase, decrease, or no change in the plasma concentration of one or both of the drugs. Because it induces hepatic enzymes, phenobarbital may enhance the hepatic clearance and decrease the clinical effectiveness of oral anticoagulants and decrease the clinical effectiveness of many other drugs.

PHENYTOIN AND FOSPHENYTOIN

Actions and Uses

Phenytoin is useful in generalized tonic-clonic, complex partial, and simple partial seizures. It is ineffective in absence, myoclonic, and atonic seizures and is not recommended for the treatment of epileptic syndromes in which absence seizures or myoclonus are present.

Available Formations

Phenytoin sodium:
    Generic: Capsules (prompt) 100 mg and 300 mg
    Dilantin® 30 mg and 100 mg.
Phenytoin (free acid):
    Dilantin® chewable tablets 50 mg
    Generic: Suspension 125 mg/5 mL (alcohol < 0.6%).
    Dilantin® (Pfizer): Suspension 125 mg/5 mL (alcohol < 0.6%).
Intravenous:
    Phenytoin 50 mg/ml
    Fosphenytoin® 75 mg/ml (same as 50 mg of phenytoin)

Absorption and Metabolism

T_{max} is 4–8 hours for prompt-release capsules and later for the extended-release preparations. Plasma protein binding is 90%. Phenytoin is eliminated almost entirely by hepatic metabolism. Small increases in dose may greatly increase the plasma concentration. Plasma concentrations of 10–20 mg/L are usually effective. However, higher or lower concentrations may sometimes be needed, and clinical outcome should determine the appropriate level for each patient.

Dosage and Administration

Oral: The dosage must be individualized according to the patient's response to the drug concentrations. Phenytoin may be administered in divided doses but does not need to be dosed more than twice daily. In adults, once-daily administration is usually sufficient to maintain plasma concentrations in the therapeutic range after a steady state has been achieved. It also improves compliance. However, once-daily dosage may not be practical in patients who tend to miss doses.

For adults, initially 300 mg daily is recommended in two divided doses; the maintenance dose is usually 4–6 mg/kg/day. Incremental increases can be made using 30-mg capsules. Formulation differences between tablet and capsules may cause problems in precise dose titration. The tablets (free acid phenytoin) contain 8% more phenytoin than the phenytoin sodium capsules. Dosing regimens for the elderly have not been well established but are usually 3–4 mg/kg/day.

Because there are differences between generic and brand, switching from one to the other should be done only with the physician's knowledge.

Side Effects

Phenytoin produces little or no sedation at concentrations below 20 mg/L. Plasma concentrations above 20 mg/L may be associated with concentration-dependent symptoms of toxicity—nystagmus, ataxia, and lethargy. However, in the absence of symptoms, doses should not be decreased if levels are above 20 mg/L.

Skin rashes occur in approximately 8% of patients within 2 weeks of initial treatment but are rarely serious. Peripheral neuropathy may develop after years of use. Mild gingival hyperplasia (thickening of the gums) may be seen on careful oral examination in 20%–50% of patients. Hirsutism (excessive hair growth) is less common.

Rare but serious idiosyncratic reactions include hepatitis, bone-marrow depression, systemic lupus erythematosus, Stevens–Johnson syndrome, and lymphadenopathy. A few cases of lymphoma and Hodgkin's disease have been reported.

Drug Interactions

Phenytoin may reduce the plasma concentration of carbamazepine, valproate, ethosuximide, and primidone by enzyme induction. Phenytoin and phenobarbital exert variable, reciprocal effects. Valproate displaces phenytoin from protein-binding sites, but inhibits metabolism. Total plasma concentrations may be decreased, but the unbound (free) sites may change little or may increase. Other drugs that may displace phenytoin include phenylbutazone, salicylates, and tolbutamide. The total plasma concentration of phenytoin may decrease, but the actual free concentration may be relatively unchanged because of the increase in the free fraction.

Drugs that significantly increase the plasma concentration of phenytoin include chloramphenicol, cimetidine, dicumarol, disulfiram, isoniazid, sulfonamids, and trimethoprim. Amiodarone, allopurinol, chlorpheniramine, and trazodone may possibly increase the plasma phenytoin concentration. Folic acid, prolonged ingestion of alcohol, and rifampin may decrease the phenytoin plasma concentration. In patients with tuberculosis, the effects of rifampin and isoniazid may cancel each other when these drugs are used with phenytoin. Certain antieoplastic agents (bleomycin, cisplatin, vinblastine) may also reduce plasma concentrations of phenytoin.

Phenytoin is a relatively potent enzyme inducer and may decrease the effectiveness of oral anticoagulants, certain antibiotics (doxycycline, rifampin, and chloramphenicol), oral contraceptives, antiarrhythmic agents (disopyramide, mexiletine, quinidine) digitoxin, analgesics (meperidine, methadone), cyclosporine, corticosteroids, and theophylline. Pharmacologically, phenytoin has been reported to impair blood pressure control by dopamine and to decrease the response to nondepolarizing skeletal muscle relaxants.

For many years, intravenous phenytoin was used for emergency treatement of seizures. However, because it may cause tissue damage, low blood pressure, or abnormal heart beats, many hospitals are using fosphenytoin instead. Fosphenytoin is safer to use and is converted to phenytoin in the body.

Pregabalin (Lyrica®)

Actions and Uses

Pregabalin binds with high affinity to a subunit of voltage-gated calcium channels located in the central nervous system. Although its precise mechanism of action is not fully understood, studies have shown it to reduce the calcium-dependent release of several neurotransmitters. It was approved by the FDA in 2005 initially for neuropathic pain, and approval for adjunct therapy for partial seizures followed within a few months. A request for use in generalized anxiety disorders has been filed.

Absorption and Eliminiation

The oral bioavailability of pregabalin is approximately 90%. Its absorption is rapid, with the time to peak concentration (T_{max}) under fasting conditions approximately 1.5 hours. Pregabalin is not bound to plasma proteins and is eliminated in the urine unchanged.

Dosage and Administration

Oral: For adults, initially 75 mg b.i.d. or 50 mg. t.i.d. (150 mg/day). Based on response and tolerability, the dose may be increased to 600 mg per day, but the rate of dose escalation has not been established. Pregabalin should be discontinued by tapering over at least 1 week. Patients with renal impairment should have their dose modified to account for reduced clearance (see PDR® or package insert).

Tablets or Capsules
   Generic: None
   Brand: Lyrica® capsules 25, 50, 75, 100, 150, 200, 225, and 300 mg.

Adverse Reactions and Precautions

The most common adverse events reported during clinical trials involved the CNS and were dose related. Dizziness was reported by 18% receiving 150 mg/day and by 38% receiving 600 mg/day. Somnolence was reported by 11% and 28%, respectively. Subjects (11%) receiving placebo reported similar symptoms. Tremor, amnesia, speech disorder, incoordination, abnormal gait, and confusion were reported by 4%–8% of subjects at rates higher than placebo. Treatment-emergent myoclonus was observed in 4% of subjects receiving 600 mg/day in studies of pregabalin for epilepsy, but was not observed in studies for pain.

Blurred vision was reported by 6% of pregabalin-treated subjects as compared to 2% for placebo, but this symptom resolved in most cases with continued dosing.

Weight gain (7% or more above baseline) was observed in 5% of the 150 mg/day subjects and 16% of the 600 mg/day during the study period. Peripheral edema independent of weight gain was observed in 5% vs. 2% for placebo.

Pregabalin has been classified as a controlled substance, schedule V (5). This was based on a study of recreational users reporting a "good effect," "high," or "likely" from the drug to a degree similar to a 30-mg dose of diazepam. In controlled studies involving more than 5,500 patients, 4% reported euphoria. Following rapid discontinuation, some patients have reported withdrawal symptoms such as insomnia, nausea, headaches, or diarrhea.

Drug Interactions

Pregabalin is not affected by a large number of drugs, including antiepileptic drugs, hypoglycemics, diuretics; and pregabalin has no effect on them.

TIAGABINE

Action and Uses

Tiagabine is a blocker of GABA reuptake, thus increasing GABA concentration in the synaptic cleft. Its major effect is to enhance the activity of GABA, the major neuroinhibitory transmitter in the central nervous system. It has been found effective for the treatment of partial seizures. It has been approved for use as adjunctive therapy in adults and children 12 years and older in the treatment of partial seizures.

Tablets
  Generic: none
  Brand: Gabitril® tablets, 4, 12, 16, and 20 mg.

Absorption and Elimination

Absorption is rapid, with a T_{max} of 45 min after an oral dose. Its half-life is 7–9 hours in volunteers, but may be 4–7 hours in patients receiving drugs that induce hepatic enzymes. It is extensively metabolized by the

CYP 3A isoform subfamily of cytochrome P-450, with only 2% of the dose excreted unchanged. Tiagabine is highly (96%) protein bound.

Doses and Administration

In adults, tiagabine should be initiated at 4 mg once a day, increased by 4 to 8 mg at weekly intervals, up to 56 mg per day. Higher doses have been used in some patients, especially those who are receiving other drugs that stimulate hepatic metabolism.

Side Effects

The most common adverse events in placebo-controlled trials were referable to the CNS and consisted of somnolence, dizziness, and difficulty with concentration. No systematic abnormalities on routine laboratory tests were noted during the studies, and no specific recommendations regarding routine monitoring have been made. Patients with a history of spike-wave abnormalities on EEG may have an exacerbation as well as clinical symptoms of lethargy or poor responsiveness.

Drug Interactions

Tiagabine has been shown not to have an effect on most drugs, including oral contraceptives. However, drugs that induce hepatic metabolism, especially phenytoin, phenobarbital and carbamazepine, significantly increase the metabolism of tiagabine and lead to the need for higher doses.

TOPIRAMATE

Action and Uses

Topiramate is a sulfamate-substituted monosaccharide that appears to have at least three distinct mechanisms of action in the central nervous system. It appears to block repetitive firing of the sodium channel, to increase the activation at $GABA_A$ receptors, and to antagonize the ability of the excitatory amino acid kainate to activate the kainate/AMPA receptor. Therefore, it has a unique profile of mechanisms covering a wide range of inhibitory and excitatory actions.

Tablets

Generic: None

Brand: Topamax® 25, 100, 200 mg

Absorption and Elimination

Absorption is rapid, with peak plasma concentrations occurring in 2 hours; bioavailability is approximately 80%, and its half-life is 21 hours. It is not extensively metabolized, with approximately 70% excreted unchanged in the urine.

Doses and Administration

In clinical trials of doses of 200, 400, 600, and 1,000 mg per day, there did not appear to be an increase of efficacy at the higher doses, but side effects were more common. The recommended daily dose for adults is 400 mg in two divided doses. Therapy should be initiated at 25 mg/day to 50 mg/day and increased by 25-mg to 50-mg increments.

Side Effects

The most common adverse reactions are somnolence, dizziness, ataxia, speech disorders, psychomotor slowing, and paresthesias. Significant kidney stones occurred in approximately 1.5% of patients during clinical trials, an incidence 2 to 4 times that expected in a similar, untreated population.

Drug Interactions

Topiramate does not appear to affect levels of other drugs. However, phenytoin and carbamazepine decrease topiramate concentrations.

VALPROATE

Actions and Uses

Valproate (valproic acid [Depakene®] and divalproex sodium [Depakote®]) control absence, myoclonic, and tonic seizures in generalized, idiopathic epilepsy. It is useful in typical absence seizures. Valproate is as effective as ethosuximide in patients with absence seizures alone and is variably effective in atypical absence seizures. Valproate is the drug of choice for patients with both absence and generalized tonic-clonic seizures.

Valproate is the drug of choice in myoclonic epilepsy, with or without generalized tonic-clonic seizures that begin in adolescence or early adulthood (juvenile myoclonic epilepsy). Valproate usually controls photosensitive myoclonus and is also effective in the treatment of benign myoclonic epilepsy, postanoxic myoclonus, and, with clonazepam, in severe progressive myoclonic epilepsy that is characterized by tonic-clonic seizures. It also may be preferred in certain stimulus-sensitive (reflex, startle) epilepsies.

Capsules
  Generic: capsules 250 mg.
  Brand: Depakene® capsules 250 mg
  Divalproex Sodium:
  Brand: Depakote® , tablets (delayed-release, DR) 125, 250, and 500 mg.
  Depakote® extended-release (ER) capsules, 125, 250, 500
  Depakote® Sprinkle, capsules 125 mg.
Syrup
  Depakene® syrup 250 mg/5 mL

Absorption and Elimination

Valproic acid is absorbed rapidly and completely in the stomach after oral administration; peak plasma concentrations usually occur within 0.5–2 hours. The delayed-release tablet preparation (DR), divalproex sodium, reaches peak plasma concentrations 3–6 hours after ingestion.

The slow-release form (ER) is absorbed slowly over many hours. Total availability of valproate is unaffected by food.

The plasma protein binding of valproate is saturable within the usual therapeutic range (approximately 90% at 75 mg/L). Usual effective plasma concentration range from 50–100 mg/L, but higher concentrations exceeding 150 mg/L may be required and tolerated in some patients. With a daily dose of more than 50 mg/kg, total plasma concentrations may not increase proportionately because both clearance and free fraction increase. Daily fluctuations in free fraction and clearance also occur as a result of displacement by free fatty acids or circadian influences.

Valproate is eliminated almost exclusively by hepatic metabolism. Its metabolic fate is complex. A variety of conjugation and oxidative processes are involved, including pathways (e.g., beta oxidation) normally reserved for endogenous fatty acids. As the dose is increased, mitochondrial beta oxidation occurs. In mitochondrial pathways, sequential use of acetyl-CoA and carnitine may interfere with intermediary metabolism. Rarely, valproate may induce secondary carnitine deficiency.

Metabolites may contribute to both antiepileptic and hepatotoxic effects. One metabolite, the 2-ene-VPA, has antiepileptic properties. Another metabolite, 2-n-propyl-4-pentenoic acid (4-ene-VPA), has been proposed as a key hepatotoxic metabolite. The half-life of valproate in adults is 12–16 hours. In patients with epilepsy receiving polytherapy, the half-life is shorter, approximately 9 hours or less in school-age children and young adolescents. Because hepatic clearance is reduced, the drug's half-life in geriatric patients is longer. Also, because of lower albumin concentrations, the free fraction may be higher in this group.

Side Effects

The incidence of gastrointestinal disturbances (nausea, vomiting, anorexia, heartburn) ranges from 6% to 45%. Symptoms are transient and rarely require drug withdrawal. Gastrointestinal discomfort may be diminished by administering the delayed-release preparation. Diarrhea, abdominal cramps, and constipation are reported occasionally. Increased appetite with weight gain is common and may be controlled by diet; but in some cases, excessive weight gain may require withdrawal of valproate.

Hand tremor, similar to benign essential tremor, is the most common neurologic side effect and occasionally is severe enough to interfere with writing. Tremor occurs more frequently with high doses and may improve with a reduction in dosage.

Sedation and drowsiness develop infrequently in patients receiving valproate alone. Conversely, central nervous system stimulation and excitement have been observed, and aggressiveness and hyperactivity are sometimes noted in children. Ataxia, headache, and stupor have been reported rarely.

Alopecia (loss of hair), thinning, or changes in hair texture occur in some patients, but these effects usually are temporary and do not require the withdrawal of the drug. Rash occurs rarely.

Valproate inhibits the secondary phase of platelet aggregation, but this is usually not clinically significant. However, patients should not receive other drugs that affect coagulation, including aspirin or coumadin. Thrombocytopenia has been observed, but its incidence is not known. Rarely, hematomas, epistaxis, and increased bleeding after surgery have been reported; and platelet function should be monitored before surgery.

A few cases of severe or fatal pancreatitis have been reported. This complication is accompanied by severe abdominal pain, vomiting, and elevated amylase.

Transient elevations of liver enzymes are common. The elevations usually are not related to serious liver dysfunction, and levels often return to normal with or without dosage adjustment. However, fatal hepatoxicity has occurred during valproate therapy. Prodromal illness characterized by muscle weakness, lethargy, anorexia, and vomiting is often present. Hepatotoxicity usually develops after an average of 2 months (range, 3 days to 6 months) of therapy.

Since 1984, hepatic fatalities associated with the use of valproate have decreased. This can be attributed to a change in the prescribing patterns for valproate, including increased use of monotherapy and decreased use in high-risk patients.

Drug Interactions

Valproate inhibits phenobarbital metabolism, and the plasma phenobarbital concentration may increase by 25% to 68% when valproate is added. This can cause marked sedation or intoxication attributable to phenobarbital.

The interaction between valproate and phenytoin is complex. Valproate displaces phenytoin from plasma albumin, which temporarily increases the ratio of free/bound drug; toxicity may result if phenytoin concentrations were high before administration of valproate. The total phenytoin plasma concentration may decrease by about 30% during the first several weeks of therapy but usually does not result in recurrence of seizures because the free phenytoin concentration does not change. However, valproate also may inhibit the biotransformation of phenytoin, which, over the next 4 to 16 weeks, produces a gradual return of total phenytoin plasma concentrations to previous values. Measurement of unbound phenytoin concentration may be useful as a means of explaining the onset of central nervous system toxicity when the total plasma phenytoin concentration is within the therapeutic range. Valproate inhibits the metabolism of carbamazepine 10,11-epoxide and of lamotrigine.

Dosage and Administration

Oral: Adults, initially 5–15 mg/kg/day; usual maintenance dose, 15–25 mg/kg/day. When used with other antiepileptic drugs, higher doses may be needed.

Children 2–12 years, initially, 10–30 mg/kg/day; maintenance dose 20–30 mg/kg/day. When used with other antiepileptic drugs that induce hepatic metabolism, the doses need to be higher. Depakote® Sprinkle may be preferable for use in children and elderly patients because it is more palatable than the syrup, can be sprinkled over food, and is slowly absorbed, which may reduce fluctuations in concentrations.

ZONISAMIDE

Actions and Uses

Zonisamide is recommended as adjunctive treatment for partial seizures in adults and children over 12 years of age. It has been available in Japan since 1990 and the experience there suggests it may be very effective for certain myoclonic syndromes.

Available Formations:
    Zonisamide
    Generic: Some doses
    Brand: Zonegran® capsules, 25, 50, 100 mg

Absorption

Zonisamide is rapidly absorbed with a T_{max} of 2–3 hours, and it has a long half-life. In human volunteers, its half-life is more than 60 hours, but this is shortened to about 30 hours when used with drugs that induce hepatic metabolism. Twice-a-day dosing is appropriate. It is predominantly metabolized by the liver, but a significant amount is excreted unchanged in the urine. Protein binding is low.

Dosage and Administration

Zonisamide can be started as 100–200 mg/day in adults, and 2–4 mg/kg/day in children. Steady state is reached in 7–10 days, and doses can be increased at 2-week intervals. Maintenance doses are usually 400–600 mg/day in adults and 4–8 mg/kg/day in children.

Side Effects

The most serious adverse event is the development of significant kidney stones in approximately 1.5% of persons in clinical trials in the United States. Interestingly, kidney stones have not been observed in Japan. Other adverse effects include somnolence, ataxia, anorexia, confusion, fatigue, and dizziness.

Drug Interactions

Zonisamide does not induce hepatic enzymes and thus does not appear to affect the metabolism of other drugs. However, in persons receiving either phenytoin or carbamazepine, the half-life of zonisamide was observed to be approximately 30 hours. On the other hand, lamotrigine may inhibit the clearance of zonisamide.

CHAPTER 5

Surgical Treatment for Epilepsy

S OME TYPES OF EPILEPSY can be helped or even cured by surgery. But before it is decided if surgery is possible, the epileptic syndrome must be correctly diagnosed. In general, people with localization-related epilepsy may be considered as possible candidates to be helped by surgery, while those with generalized epilepsy may not. The most important aspect in the decision process, then, is carefully identifying the area or areas from which the seizures are coming, and then locating the important areas of brain function such as speech, memory, motor control, etc. Only when all of this information is carefully analyzed can the epilepsy team develop a risk/benefit evaluation. The final decision about surgery should be made by the person with epilepsy but only after the possible outcomes are clearly understood.

When a brain tumor is found to be the cause of the epilepsy there is often a great deal of worry and the initial impulse is to operate immediately. However, many tumors that cause epilepsy are slow-growing or stable (benign). Seizures usually arise from brain tissue next to the tumor and its removal may cause problems. Localizing the origin of the seizures is important because then one operation can be designed to both remove the tumor and control the seizures. If the tumor is close to important areas such as memory, speech, or motor function, and surgery might damage these, it may be better to delay surgery.

On the other hand, some persons with epilepsy, or their advocates, are sometimes overly reluctant to proceed with surgery even though there is a good possibility of a "cure," In all cases, the epilepsy treatment team should be sensitive to the emotional issues involved. A person who has invested a great deal of time and money into the surgical evaluation and treatment will experience a great deal of frustration if the evaluation and treatment do not result in surgery or cure. Paradoxically, an excellent outcome of freedom from seizures may also be accompanied by emotional difficulties. Many persons who have had frequent seizures have not developed educational and socialization skills to fully integrate into employment and personal activities immediately after surgery. Also, they may lose some of their financial support systems such as disability payments. Although they now are free from seizures, their own expectations and those of others may not be met quickly. It is not unusual for there to be a gap of a few years between completely successful surgery and full reintegration into society. An experienced epilepsy treatment team is aware of this phenomenon and will provide support during the post-operative period.

Determining whether a person should have surgery should be done in a stepwise process, with tests performed in logical order as results from tests become available. The first step is to determine if a person has epilepsy that has not been controlled after two or three AEDs have been tried using the correct drugs and dosages. If the epilepsy is localization related, referral to an epilepsy center should be considered. There are a number of epilepsy centers in the United States, and information about them can be obtained from a neurologist or from the National Association of Epilepsy Centers (call 952-525-4507).

TYPES OF SURGERY

There are different types of surgery. Some types involve cutting the brain, and other types involve placing devices.

Surgeries that involve cutting include the following:

- Temporal lobectomy is the removal or part of or all of one temporal lobe. This is the most common and successful type of surgery for epilepsy.
- Topectomy is the removal of the surface layers of the brain (cortex).
- Lesionectomy is the removal of a tumor, haemartoma, or other clearly defined lesion.

- Hemispherectomy is the removal of half of the brain.
- Corpus callostomy is cutting the fibers (axons) connecting the two halves of the brain.
- Subpial transaction is cutting the fibers (axons) connecting surface regions of the brain (cortex).

Surgeries that involve implanting devices include the following:

- Vagus nerve stimulator is a pacemaker-like device used to stimulate the vagus nerve in the neck.
- Direct brain stimulation involves placing a stimulating device directly into the brain. This may become available in a few years.

PHASE I: INPATIENT PRESURGICAL EVALUATION

The goal of this evaluation is to record seizures to further clarify the types of seizures and their sites of origin. This involves video-EEG monitoring 24 hours per day. Sometimes special electrodes, such as the sphenoidal electrode, are used. These are small recording wires placed through the jaw muscle to be close to the middle part of the temporal lobe.

Often, AEDs are reduced or eliminated to increase the number of seizures. However, some people have almost daily seizures, and medicines do not need to be reduced. The length of stay depends on how often seizures occur, but the average time is 5 to 10 days. The purpose is to record partial seizures but to avoid generalized tonic-clonic seizures, so rescue medicines are used to slow down seizures if they begin to happen too quickly. Orders for these medicines (such as lorazepam, diazepam intramuscular fosphenytoin, or intravenous valproate) are written at the time of admission. Nursing care is designed to prevent any injury and also to provide observations such as ability to follow commands, to remember and recall things, and the ability to speak during seizures.

Neuropsychological testing is crucial in helping identify local areas of dysfunction. For example, deficits in verbal memory implicate the left temporal lobe. Because a temporal lobectomy should be avoided if the remaining temporal lobe cannot maintain memory function, the intracarotid Amytal® test (Wada test) is critical. During this test, first one and then the other carotid artery is injected with a short-acting drug such as Amytal®, resulting in arrest of cerebral function of the injected area for 10–15 minutes. Speech and memory testing is performed, and it is thus possible to determine the approximate functional capacity of the opposite hemisphere in the absence of the injected hemisphere, providing an assessment of postoperative functioning.

SPECT and PET Scans

Because an MRI scan only shows the structure of the brain, not its function, other tests have been developed to help locate areas from which seizures arise. Usually, the areas from which seizures arise are not working normally and use less glucose (blood sugar) and oxygen than areas which are working normally. During a seizure, however, the areas involved in the seizure are working harder than other areas and accordingly are using more glucose and oxygen.

An interictal (i.e., between seizures) SPECT scan will show less activity. During a seizure, however, those areas of the brain are more active and an ictal (during the seizure) scan can be very helpful. However, to obtain this type of scan a small amount of a tracer material must be injected into a vein as soon as possible after the start of a seizure, preferably within seconds. The findings of the ictal SPECT scan can then be compared with the interictal scan. This will highlight the area of the seizure because the low interictal activity and the high ictal activity will stand out more from the normal activity. Unfortunately, getting an ictal SPECT can only be done in the hospital and may require repeated tries to get the best ictal scan.

A PET (positron emission tomography) scan uses glucose labeled with a positive electron instead of a negative (usual) electron. Positrons are antimatter, and when they collide with an electron, they turn into energy in the form of a gamma ray pulse. Areas of the brain that are less active use less glucose and therefore give off fewer gamma rays. The PET scan is easier to do than a SPECT scan, so a PET scan is often done first. If it does not give a good location but hints at one, a SPECT scan is then considered.

PHASE II EVALUATION

Sometimes the Phase I evaluation shows that the seizures seem to be coming from an area that may be close to an important area such as speech. The electrodes used for the EEG are on the skin and are about 1 inch away from the brain. They are also usually a few inches apart. Therefore, they can locate the seizure onset area only to within a few inches of the exact location. If the location seems to be near the motor strip, speech area, or other important region, direct recording from the brain may be necessary. In the past, this was done in the operating room with the patient awake under local anesthesia. Today, however, this is rarely done. A better way is the use of electrical contacts placed directly on the surface of the brain (Figure 5-1). These electrodes are 1 centimeter (less than 1/2-inch) apart. Each electrode is used to record brain signals; and during a seizure, the location and spread of the abnormal electrical activity can be mapped.

Placement of the grid (group of electrodes) is done at the beginning of phase II (Figure 5-2). A bone flap is lifted and the grid is gently placed on the surface of the brain. The bone flap is then put back, and the wires from the grid come out of a small hole in the bone and out of the skin. These wires are connected by a cable to the recording equipment. Usually, the recording and stimulation lasts for one week. The general anesthesia wears off in a few hours, and the usual activities of wakefulness such as

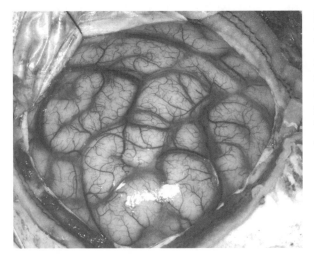

FIGURE 5-1

The brain exposed for surgery. This has been done by removing a rectangular piece of skull bone (bone flap) which can be replaced after surgery.

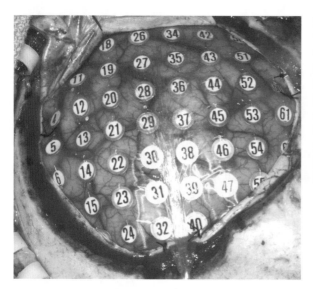

FIGURE 5-2

A grid made of soft plastic with recording contacts has been placed on the surface of the brain. The bone flap will then be replaced, and recording of seizures will be made.

reading, eating, and talking can be followed. Some patients feel very little discomfort for the week of recording, but others have headaches and do not feel well.

These electrodes can also be used to map the location of critical areas of function. For example, during stimulation, a small electrical pulse is sent to an electrode, and the patient's response is carefully observed. At the end of the phase II evaluation, the areas of seizure activity and the location of vital functions have been mapped. The epilepsy treatment team can then decide how best to control epilepsy with little or no injury to vital areas. For example, if seizures are coming from electrodes 12, 13, 20, and 21, and speech is at 30, 31, 38, 39, 46, and 47, the surgeon can remove 12, 13, 20, but may want to leave 21 because it is close to the speech area. This would be discussed with the patient as a situation where a reduction but not complete elimination of seizures would be the most likely outcome.

When the recording is complete and the epilepsy treatment team and the patient have decided what to do, another operation is performed. During this, the surgeon lifts up the bone flap, removes the grid, carefully noting the areas of brain under each electrode, and then removes the tissue identified as the source of the seizures, replaces the bone flap, and closes the skin incision.

Recovery from this step is 4 to 6 days.

Strips and Depth Electrodes

Although grids are the most commonly used recording electrodes, others can be used in special circumstances. Strip electrodes are single rows of electrodes, usually four electrodes in one strip, one centimeter apart, which can be placed over areas too small for a grid. They can be placed through a small hole, avoiding the need for a bone flap. An alternative to using grids or strips is placing depth electrodes. These are long, stiff wires with contact points similar in function to the electrodes on the grid. These pass through brain tissue to get to the area to be studied. They are most often used when the area of interest is in the middle of the temporal lobe.

Temporal Lobectomy

The most common surgically approachable epilepsy syndrome is mesial temporal sclerosis. A typical case includes a febrile convulsion during the first few years of life. Seizures may start in the teen years, usually as complex partial seizures, but also may first come to attention as a secondarily generalized tonic-clonic seizure. Treatment with AEDs is usually effective in blocking the generalized tonic-clonic seizures, but complex partial seizures may continue. An electroencephalogram (EEG) often shows interictal spikes (electrical signals happening between seizures) arising from one or both temporal lobes. An MRI scan, if done properly, may show small changes in one or both temporal lobes.

Neuropsychological testing may show a decrease in memory functioning. This can be especially useful if it shows that visual memory (usually the right temporal lobe) or verbal memory (left temporal lobe) is impaired. PET and SPECT scans may also be useful. Intracarotid Amytal testing is often very helpful in demonstrating that one temporal lobe is not working and that its removal can be done with little harm to memory. Sometimes, if the damage to one temporal lobe is done in the first few years of life, the other temporal lobe can take over both verbal and visual memory. This is the best situation for surgery.

If all of these tests (EEG, MRI, neuropsychological testing, and Wada) point to one temporal lobe, the outcome can be very favorable.

Approximately 80% of persons with this profile may be seizure-free after surgery, and suffer little, if any, side effects. Some may also be taken off AEDs three or four years after surgery if they have had no further seizures and their EEG is normal. However, the goal is complete freedom from seizures, not discontinuation of AEDs. Many persons are being treated with two or more AEDs, and it is possible to eliminate one after surgery in almost all cases. Most of the rest of those having a temporal lobectomy have a marked decrease in the number of seizures, a few have no change, and rarely are seizures made worse. Many people find that with their seizures eliminated or reduced, their mental functioning improves because seizures are no longer interfering with mental activity.

Most of the risks are from the surgical procedure. These should be fully discussed with the neurosurgeon. The most serious risks are stroke, bleeding, infection, and complications from anesthesia. These are rarely fatal. Overall, the risk of serious complications is approximately 3%. There is no good way of predicting who will have a complication, and surgery done by even the most experienced neurosurgeons is not risk-free. Removal of a temporal lobe that contains the hippocampus may affect memory functioning. Also, because most people have speech function in the left brain in the back part of the temporal lobe, speech may be affected.

TOPECTOMY, LESIONECTOMY, AND SUBPIAL TRANSECTION

If an area from which seizures arise can be identified from mapping after a phase II evaluation, removal of that region is called a topectomy. Because the area of the brain associated with producing seizures cannot always be completely mapped, the probability of complete freedom from seizures is often less than from temporal lobectomy, in the range of 50%–70%. Lesionectomy refers to removing the lesion, such as a tumor. With a lesionectomy, if the lesion is small and easily removed, the chance for seizure freedom may be greater than with a topectomy.

In addition to the risks of stroke, bleeding, and infection, topectomy and lesionectomy carry the risk of damaging whichever function is close. If near the motor strip, weakness or paralysis of a hand, arm, leg, or face is possible. If near visual cortex or visual projections, alteration of vision is possible. If near the speech area, alteration of speech can be a complication.

Sometimes the area of the epilepsy is in the same area as a vital function. In these situations, a procedure called multiple subpial transaction can be done. In this procedure, the neurosurgeon will make a series of cuts vertical to the surface of the brain, hoping to disconnect the epileptic neurons from normal neurons, allowing them to work more normally without interference. Often, multiple subpial transaction is done with a topectomy or lesionectomy, the former removing abnormal tissue while the subpial transection may help control seizures while minimizing the side effects.

Hemispherectomy

In this procedure, half of the brain, or a hemisphere, is removed. This surgery, while drastic, can be very effective in children who have very serious damage to half of their brain from a stroke, malformation, or other cause. Because children with these conditions have very frequent and severe seizures, risk of death from frequent seizures or very delayed development is a reality. With EEG, MRI, PET, and SPECT scans, the affected hemisphere can usually be identified. Children with these conditions usually already have hemiplegia (paralysis of the body side opposite the side of the damaged hemisphere). Removal of the motor cortex causes little change. Except for the usual risks of surgery, this drastic operation often causes no further changes. Remarkably, stopping or reducing seizures often leads to greatly improved learning and development even though a large part of the brain has been removed.

Corpus Callosotomy

Some persons with very severe epilepsy have damage in both sides of the brain, and therefore cannot have any of the aforementioned procedures. However, because seizures on one side of the brain can cross over to the other and excite the seizure-prone areas there, cutting the connections can be helpful The two sides of the brain communicate with each other with neurons from one side sending axons to the other side through a bundle of axons. This group of axons forms a structure called the corpus collosum. This bundle of fibers can be cut surgically, isolating one side of the brain from the other. This operation is most successful for stopping very rapid generalized seizures, which lead to drop seizures. These are associated with falls and serious head injury. Persons with this type of seizure often need to wear helmets because they may have many drop seizures each day. This surgery is often successful in markedly decreasing the number of drop seizures, but other seizure types such as partial motor or complex partial seizures are not affected. The risks of this operation include stroke, bleeding, infection, and complications from anesthesia. Surprisingly, it has little effect on other functions. However, this may be difficult to judge because most people who are candidates for this type of surgery have the Lennox–Gastaut syndromes or similar conditions affecting intellectual functioning. Unlike the other surgical procedures, the recovery time after corpus callosotomy may be many weeks and require physical therapy.

THE VAGUS NERVE STIMULATOR

The vagus nerve stimulator (VNS) may be a treatment option for patients who have intractable epilepsy but who are not candidates for surgical options. A complete phase I evaluation should be done before considering the use of a vagus nerve stimulator to be sure that a more definitive surgery is not available. Overall, the vagus nerve stimulator can reduce seizures by about 50%. A few people out of a hundred will have complete control.

The vagus nerve stimulator is flat, round, and about the size of a cardiac pacemaker. It contains a battery pack, a computer chip, and connecting wire. Similar to a cardiac pacemaker, the VNS is implanted in the chest under the clavicle(collar bone), and the leads at the end of the connecting wire are attached to the vagus nerve on the left side of the neck (Figure 5-3). With this device, the vagus nerve can be stimulated

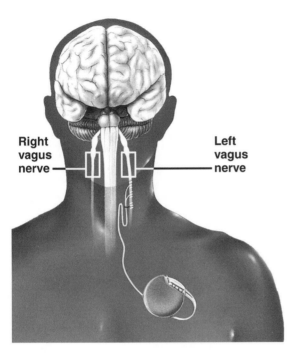

Right vagus nerve

Left vagus nerve

FIGURE 5-3

The vagus nerve stimulator looks like a cardiac pacemaker. It is placed under the skin over the left chest wall muscle. Wires are then tunneled under the skin and wrapped around the vagus nerve.

approximately every 5 minutes for about 30 seconds. The stimulation parameters(settings) can be adjusted by an external magnetic device controlled by a laptop computer in the physician's office. In addition, an external magnet can be applied by the patient or a caregiver during a seizure to stop the convulsion.

Patients who experience auras warning them of an impending seizure can stop or shorten the length of the seizure by activating the VNS. This is done by holding a magnet over the pocket of skin that hides the VNS. Based on two double-blind studies demonstrating efficacy and safety, the Food and Drug Administration (FDA) approved the VNS for the treatment of epilepsy in 1997. The surgery is relatively minor, and complications are few. During stimulation, the patient's voice may be hoarse, or there may be minor pain. Infections are rare but may require removal of the device. Direct surgery is more effective than VNS so the option of temporal lobectomy or other surgical procedures should be explored before using a VNS.

DIRECT BRAIN STIMULATION

Because the brain is in some ways is similar to the heart, the concept that seizures can be controlled by stimulation of the brain has developed. Studies involving patients are now being done, but it is too early to know how well this approach will work. One concept is to use totally implanted seizure detection devices linked to stimulation devices that will be activated to block seizures. Other concepts would be to deliver AEDs directly to the area of the brain when seizures appear to be starting.

CHAPTER 6

Epilepsy and Women's Issues

Approximately half of all persons with epilepsy are women. It is well-known that women with epilepsy have a number of special issues to consider. These include birth control, pregnancy, hormone replacement therapy, menopause, and change in seizures during menstrual cycles. Hormones can influence epilepsy. Estrogen appears to make the brain more likely to have seizures, while progesterone may make it less likely to have a seizure. The changing balance of hormones throughout life may complicate the treatment of epilepsy in women. It is speculated that the onset of epilepsy in many women during the teenage years is related to the onset of menses. What happens to epilepsy during and after menopause is not well understood.

Seizures and Menstrual Cycles

Many women experience seizures related to their cycles. This has been called catamenial epilepsy. As many as one-third of women with epilepsy have an increase in their seizures during parts of their cycle. Although this is a well-known phenomenon, very little is understood about how or why it happens or how to best treat it. Some physicians have reported that the use of progesterone in various forms may help prevent seizures during the cycle. However, many women experience troublesome side-effects from progesterone and give up using it. Also, use of progesterone does not always work well to stop seizures. Some physicians have prescribed acetazolamide (Diamox) during periods. This works sometimes, but again, exact timing of use can be uncertain. If there is a very strong relationship between times in the cycle and seizures, these treatments can be tried.

Birth Control

There are a number of options for birth control, and what is best for a woman with epilepsy depends on many issues. Barrier methods have the advantage of not involving use of hormones, but are often less convenient. Hormonal contraceptives involve the use of estrogen or progesterone, or both. Although there is a theoretical risk of estrogen exacerbating seizures, this does not seem to be a problem for most women. Some women like to use the injectable hormone medroxyprogesterone, which needs to be given only once every three months (DepoProvera). Some women have noticed that their seizure control is actually better when using this method.

Because both hormones and AEDs are metabolized in the liver, there can be changes in the patterns of elimination. Many AEDs induce (stimulate) the liver enzymes that eliminate hormones. When a woman is using these AEDs, the amount of hormone in the contraceptive pills must be increased. Although the amount of hormones taken is larger, because the liver eliminates more of the hormone, the overall effect is that of taking a "normal" hormone-containing pill. Not using the appropriate oral contraceptive could result in unplanned pregnancies. Of the drugs used to treat epilepsy, phenobarbitol, primidone, phenytoin, carbamazepine, and oxcarbazepine have the strongest effect on hormonal contraceptives. All the other AEDs have a minor or no effect.

Hormones may afffect the concentration of some AEDs. Estrogen can have a large effect on the concentrations of lamotrigine. A recent study showed that women taking the 21-day-on, 7-day-off oral contraceptives had their lamotrigine change dramatically. When the oral contraceptive is given for 21 days, lamotrigine levels decrease to half of what the concentration was before the hormone. Then, when no hormone is given for the 7 days, the lamotrigine levels double, back to the no-hormone level. It appears that estrogen is the major factor causing this dramatic change in levels. Women receiving lamotrigine should probably choose a form of contraception that does not cycle, is mostly progesterone, or instead use nonhormonal methods.

PREGNANCY

Although women with epilepsy face greater risks in childbearing than women with no chronic illnesses, these risks are not great enough (with a few exceptions) to preclude having a family. The woman and her partner have the responsibility of deciding whether or not to have children after they have obtained appropriate medical information about risks. Unfortunately, there is much misinformation about actual risks, and many women with epilepsy have been told they should not have children. Often overlooked in this decision are risks other than epilepsy, which may have much greater consequences on pregnancy outcome than seizures or antiepileptic drugs.

There are many questions raised by women with epilepsy (Figure 6-1), including:

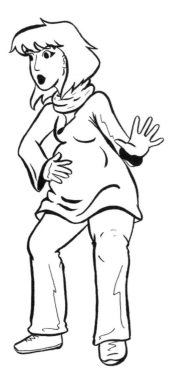

FIGURE 6-1

I'm pregnant. Now what about my epilepsy?

- What are the effects of pregnancy on the frequency of seizures?
- What are the effects of seizures on the developing child?
- What are the effects of antiepileptic drugs on the growth and development of the baby?
- Are there changes in AED levels during pregnancy?
- Are there problems with labor and delivery?
- Is breast-feeding possible?
- What is the ability of a mother with epilepsy to care for her child?

SEIZURE FREQUENCY DURING PREGNANCY

In a review of studies describing 2,165 pregnancies, 24% had an increase in seizures, 23% a decrease, and 53% no change. The best predictor of seizure frequency during pregnancy was seizure frequency before pregnancy. Almost all patients who had more than one seizure per month had an increase in seizures during pregnancy, whereas women having less than one seizure every 9 months did not experience an increase in seizures during pregnancy. Psychological stress factors, such as anxiety leading to lack of sleep, may be important in lowering resistance to seizures. Many studies have shown that the major cause for increased seizures during pregnancy is that women do not take all of their medicine out of fear of harming the developing baby. However, seizures cause much more harm. If medicines are missed, one can develop a series of seizures called status epilepticus (Chapter 11). In one report of 29 cases of status epilepticus during pregnancy, 9 women died, as did 14 of the babies.

Balancing risk from medications against risk from increased seizures is a tough decision (Figure 6-2) and requires the exercise of careful judgment based on the most current information.

EFFECT OF SEIZURES ON THE DEVELOPING CHILD

There are a number of reports in the medical literature indicating that tonic-clonic seizures during pregnancy can be very harmful to the baby. In one case, a 28-year-old woman missed several doses of medication,

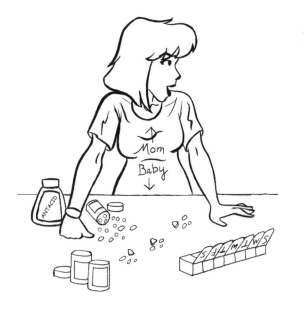

FIGURE 6-2

Tough decisions.

had generalized tonic-clonic seizures at weeks 19, 28, and 33, and delivered a stillborn baby. Seizures, by increasing intrauterine pressure and other changes can cause the fetal heart rate to slow down considerably.

While case reports are dramatic, population-based studies give a better picture of the extent of the problem. The Collaborative Perinatal Project of the National Institutes of Health studied women selected to represent the general population. In this sample, approximately 0.4% (4 out of 1,000) of women had one or more generalized tonic-clonic seizures during pregnancy. The rate of stillborn births in women with seizures (not including eclampsia) was 5.14%, significantly higher than the 2.4% in women with epilepsy but who had no seizures during the pregnancy. Head size that was in the lower 2% of the population was significantly greater in women who had a seizure during pregnancy. The rate for mixed cerebral palsy and for mental retardation was also greater. Thus, it is evident from this large study that seizures occurring during pregnancy can impair fetal development and cause stillbirth.

Complex partial seizures may result in accidents or injuries that may harm the mother and thus indirectly harm the developing child. An example would be major burns suffered by a pregnant woman as a consequence of a complex partial seizure. Such a situation would subject the developing child to all of the physiological changes that occur with extensive third-degree burns and to the risks from the multiple drugs used to treat them. Therefore, the goal of therapy should be to achieve control of all seizures during pregnancy.

BIRTH DEFECTS FROM ANTIEPILEPTIC DRUGS

There has been a great deal of confusion about the risks of birth defects in children born to mothers with epilepsy. This is because many of the reports in the medical literature about this topic during the last 30 years studied too few pregnancies or selected women not representative of the normal population. In evaluating information in medical reports, you should ask the following:

- were there enough persons in the study?
- were there other factors which could explain the results?

In general, older studies with small numbers of subjects have shown higher rates of malformations than more recent studies with thousands of patients and sampling strategies that avoid errors. Birth defects normally happen in approximately 2 to 3 out of 100 pregnancies. In order to prove that an AED increases this risk, many hundreds of pregnancies in women taking an AED must be compared to women in similar circumstances not taking these drugs. The women with epilepsy and those used for comparison should represent the overall population.

Many people are troubled about women with epilepsy having babies, but do not consider this to be a major problem with other medical conditions such as diabetes. However, the results from a large study showed that the risk is much higher in women with diabetes. In a study of 62,265 births in Australia, 3.4% (or 34 in 1,000) children born to women without diabetes or epilepsy had birth defects, compared to 3.7% born to women with epilepsy and 8.4% of children born to mothers with diabetes.[1]

---

[1] Stanley FJ, Prescott PK, Johnston R, et al: Congenital malformations in infants of mothers with diabetes and epilepsy in Western Australia, 1980–1982. *Med J. Aust* 1985; 143:440–442.

There are a number of things that can contribute to birth defects, which have nothing to do with epilepsy or AEDs. These include smoking, drinking alcohol, using street drugs, not taking vitamins, and not getting good prenatal care. Also, the risk of birth defects increases with the age of the mother. In addition, there may be genetic and geographical factors. Many older studies did not control for these variables. One notorious study examined only women from a poor district in Seattle and reported that use of an antiepileptic drug caused significant problems—but the investigator did not consider that these women also had many other problems. Since then, other large, controlled studies have not supported these findings; but this misleading study is still used to discourage women with epilepsy.

Recent large studies have shown that birth defects are related to specific AEDs; some have a higher risk than others. One of the most careful studies was done in the Netherlands. It studied women for a period of more than 20 years, and evaluated 1,411 children born to women with epilepsy and 2,000 births to women without epilepsy (the control group) from the same hospitals and of the same age. Thus, factors such as difference in medical care, nutrition, living conditions, and age were eliminated. In this study, 29 of the 2,000 children born to mothers without epilepsy (1.45%) had major malformations (Table 6-1).

Of the common antiepileptic drugs used alone, valproate had the highest risk, with carbamazepine the next riskiest. Interestingly, phenytoin used alone did not appear to be associated with an increased risk. Other studies have suggested that phenytoin may pose a risk, but these studies included many patients who were on more than one AED. Use of more than one antiepileptic drug increased the risk; and the more types of drugs used, the greater the risk. Little data is available regarding human teratogenicity (birth defects) of the newer AEDs. However, animal studies of teratogenicity have not shown major problems. More large-scale studies are in progress. So far, these studies have shown that phenobarbital may be associated with the most problems and the newer AEDs have the least.

After you study Table 6-1, you may wonder why any physician would recommend any AED or combination with a risk ratio greater than one. The main reasons are seizure control and side effects. For

Table 6-1   Antiepileptic Drugs and Major Malformations Observed in a Large Study of 2,000 Controls and 1,411 Children Born to Mothers with Epilepsy Using Antiepileptic Drugs. (Monotherapy is use of AED by itself, polytherapy is two or more AEDs .*)

Group	Number in study	Number of children with malformations	Percent of children with malformations	Risk ratio*
Control	2,000	29	1.45	1.0
Monotherapy				
Phenytoin	151	1	0.6	0.5
Carbamazepine	376	14	3.7	2.6
Valproate	159	9	5.7	4.1
Polytherapy				
Phenytoin	209	6	2.9	2.0
Benzodiazepines	106	6	5.7	4.1
Carbamazepine	225	12	5.3	3.8
Valproate	136	8	5.9	3.7
Caffeine	75	5	6.7	4.9
Any 2 AEDs	342	16	4.7	3.3
Any 3 AEDs	91	4	4.4	3.1
Any 4 AEDs	52	4	7.7	5.9

* Samrén E, Van Duijn C, Christiaens G, et al: Antiepileptic drug regimens and major congenital abnormalities in the offspring. *Ann Neurol* 1999; 46 (5):739–746. Monotherapy is AED used by itself. Polytherapy is used of an AED with other AEDs. The risk ratio is the measure of how much worse the risk for the AED-using group is compared to the control group. A risk ratio of 1 means that the control group and the AED group are the same; that is, there is no increased risk. A risk ratio of 2 means that the AED group is twice as likely to have children with malformations as the control group, and a risk ratio of 4 means that the AED group is four times as likely to have children with malformations as the control group.

example, valproate has a risk ratio of 4.1, but for many women with juvenile myoclonic epilepsy, it is the only AED effective in controlling seizures (and seizures may do more harm than the drug). In addition, if there is a small normal risk, increasing the risk by four-fold still is a small risk. Thus, for valproate, if 100 women were taking it during pregnancy, approximately 92 would have no major malformations.

In addition to concern about major malformations, there has been some concern about minor malformations. Many of these are most noticeable at birth and then become less obvious with the passage of time. Examples are strabismus ("crooked eyes"), ptosis (eyelids not opening fully), ocular hypertelorism (eyes far apart), broadened fingernail bed, small fingernails, hernias, unusual fingerprints, and minor deformities of the feet. There are reports that have associated all of the older AEDs with these minor malformations. However, carefully done studies including children born to women without epilepsy also find many of these malformations, but at a lower rate.

Overall, the vast majority of women with epilepsy have normal children, and risks can be reduced with good planning.

Every woman has her own level of risk tolerance: some want absolutely no risk, while others wish to have children regardless of risk. Physicians must be knowledgeable about the risks and benefits of each drug and then counsel each family appropriately. The final decision to have children should be left to the woman, but physicians have the obligation to make sure that the woman clearly understands the issues. Blanket statements that women with epilepsy should not have children are not appropriate, and complete avoidance of an AED that may significantly reduce seizures is also not logical. Not controlling seizures during pregnancy may be worse than using an AED with some risk.

CHANGES IN AED LEVELS DURING PREGNANCY

Drug absorption. Gastric tone and motility are reduced during pregnancy, resulting in delayed emptying of the stomach. Antacids are frequently prescribed during pregnancy. Dimethicone, a common constituent of antacids, reduces phenytoin absorption by 71%, and kaolin reduces it by 60%, whereas magnesium trisilicate has a negligible effect. Nausea and vomiting are other symptoms during pregnancy that affect drug ingestion and absorption, especially during the first trimester.

Metabolism. Pregnancy prompts changes in almost every aspect of metabolism. A number of changes occur in the liver, and these may affect drug metabolism. The rising concentrations of steroids increase the capacity for hydroxylation, and these substances are competitive inhibitors of microsomal oxidases for some drugs and may reduce their elimination.

SPECIFIC ANTIEPILEPTIC DRUGS

Carbamazepine. Although decreases in total plasma concentrations are not as great as for phenytoin, carbamazepine levels have been shown in a number of studies to decrease during pregnancy. Evaluation of carbamazepine is complicated by the fact that it is an active metabolite, carbamazepine 0,11-epoxide. Because this metabolite has been shown to have antiepileptic effects as well as toxicity and teratogenicity, decisions regarding management of patients on carbamazepine should consider the concentrations of both the parent compound and the epoxide.

Carbamazepine is absorbed relatively slowly and there is wide variability in its bioavailability. This may stem from its very slow dissolution rate into the gastrointestinal fluid. Alterations of carbamazepine absorption during pregnancy have been demonstrated.

Carbamazepine is approximately 75% protein bound, 25% unbound. No significant changes of carbamazepine binding during pregnancy have been reported.

Lamotrigine levels decrease very significantly during pregnancy, more than those of any other AED. One study in which women at one clinic had levels drawn before, during, and after pregnancy found that some women had as much as a 200% increase in elimination, and needed more than double their dose to keep the levels similar to the pre-pregnancy levels. Other women had a smaller change. The elimination rate returned to pre-pregnancy values within weeks after delivery. Women being treated with lamotrigine should have their levels checked before pregnancy and as soon as they become pregnant. The physician should change the lamotrigine dose based on the decrease in the levels, using an equation published in the neurological literature.[2] Levels should be checked during pregnancy as well, to make other adjustments if needed. After delivery the pre-pregnancy dose should be used again. Otherwise the levels may get too high and side effects such as dizziness, tiredness, and loss of energy may appear.

---

[2]Tran TA, Leppik IE, Blesi K, Sathanandan ST, Remmel R, et al. Lamotrigine clearance during pregnancy. *Neurology* 2002 59(2):251–55.)

So far, there is no definite evidence that the levels of other newer AEDs change during pregnancy. Because studies have not yet been done, it is a good idea to have levels checked.

Phenytoin concentrations may decrease significantly during pregnancy. Levels of phenytoin during pregnancy have been reported to be decreased by as much as 50%. The fetal liver and placenta are both able to metabolize drugs, which may account for some of the phenytoin eliminated. One large study showed phenytoin elimination increased gradually during the first 32 weeks of pregnancy, reached twice the preconception value during the last 8 weeks, and began to return to normal during the 12-week period after pregnancy. Malabsorption may also play a role in decreased levels, especially if certain antacids are used.

In normal women 8–15 weeks pregnant, phenytoin binding measured in vitro is within normal limits. However, women progressing beyond the 16th week of gestation have decreased binding of phenytoin to plasma proteins. This change in binding persists for at least 5 days after delivery and returns to normal 5 to 7 weeks postpartum

Valproate. Decreased concentrations during pregnancy have been noted. In one study, the concentration of valproate by the third trimester was found to have fallen to less than one-half of the first trimester value.

Valproate is metabolized to a number of compounds, with the two main metabolites being the 2-ene and the 3-keto. There is some suggestion that during pregnancy valproate metabolism may be significantly altered. There is an increased elimination of valproate during the third trimester, which may have multiple mechanisms. Valproate is highly plasma protein bound. Its plasma protein binding is significantly decreased in pregnant women

LABOR AND DELIVERY

Overall, there may be a small increase in the usual complications of labor and delivery in women with epilepsy, but these can be minimized by the appropriate obstetrical care. A major concern is having seizures

Table 6-2   Tips for Managing Conception, Pregnancy, and Delivery

Before you get pregnant:
- Find out about risks.
- Use the best medicine for seizure control and pregnancy outcome.
- Find out if continued medication is needed
  - may discontinue if seizure free for two or more years and risk for further seizures is low;
  - do not discontinue medication if epilepsy syndrome suggests continued need for treatment
- Reduce medicines to one drug if possible.
- Start folic acid.
- Eliminate other risk factors (smoking, drugs, alcohol).

After conception:
- Do not change antiepileptic medication without consulting a specialist.
- Get prenatal care.
- Take vitamins, including folic acid.
- Check blood levels every trimester and change doses as needed.
- Evaluate for neural tube defects at 12-16 weeks (ultrasound, alpha-fetoprotein, amniocentesis).
- Check antiepileptic drug levels prior to delivery and increase doses if needed.

After delivery:
- Check levels and adjust doses.

during labor and delivery. This is rare. However, home delivery is not recommended for women with epilepsy.

Infant Care

Breast-feeding has been an issue of great debate. There is much misinformation about it. Nearly all AEDs are transferred in breast milk to some degree. The amount of phenytoin in breast milk is only 18% of the amount in blood, for phenobarbital 36%, primidone 70%, carbamazepine 41%, and only 4%–5% for valproate. This means that actually very little of the AED is in the breast milk and the infant receives a very small dose. The doses an infant receives are much lower than those they are exposed to before birth and breast feeding is encouraged (Figure 6-3). Women are often told that they cannot breast feed if taking AEDs, but nothing could be further from the truth!

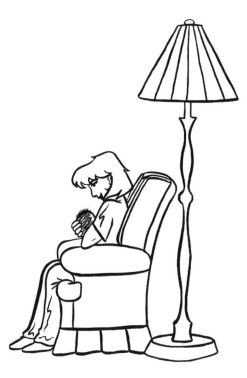

FIGURE 6-3

Breastfeeding is safe.

Women with epilepsy can safely be mothers, but some common sense things should be considered (Figure 6-4). The most common issues are those involving safety of the infant in case of seizures. The following common sense steps should be taken:

- Always have help when bathing the baby.
- Diaper changes should be done in a place where the child can be secured so that it cannot roll off the surface.
- The baby should be put on the floor if there is a warning of an oncoming seizure.

Injuries to children of mothers with epilepsy have been very rare and probably are less common than in mothers without epilepsy because extra care is taken.

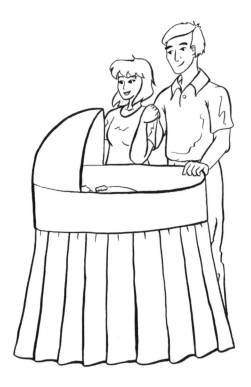

FIGURE 6-4

Caring for the baby is a joint effort.

Menopause

There have been very few studies of epilepsy in women during and after menopause. Some studies have detected an increase in seizures during this phase, but others have shown just the opposite. There is no evidence that using hormone replacement therapy has any definite effect on seizures after menopause. However, because so few studies have been done on this subject, future information may change these views.

CHAPTER 7

Epilepsy
in the Elderly

SETTING THE RETIREMENT age at 70 years was done in the 1890s by Otto
von Bismarck's cabinet in Germany. Thus, a government-sponsored
retirement system, with benefits starting at age 70, when the lifespan
was 48 years, was established. There was no medical basis for setting the
age of retirement; rather, it was a political decision. Later, the retirement
age was decreased to 65 in most countries. Research on aging has shown
that there is no uniform process of aging, so the definitions used admin-
istratively may not be useful for treatment.

For a meaningful definition of "elderly," subdivisions have been suggested. These are the "young old", 65–74 years; the "middle old", 75–84
years; and "oldest old", 85 years and older. However, on closer examination, even these subdivisions are not adequate. Many elderly are generally healthy, even in their later years. On the other hand, some elderly have handicapping medical problems, and some, especially in nursing
homes, are frail. Obviously drug side effects, efficacy, absorption and
other factors will differ greatly between a 93-year-old healthy person as
compared with a 68-year-old frail person. Thus, to add precision to the
elderly, the categorization in Table 7-1 is useful.

The likelihood of developing epilepsy begins to increase after age 50,
and the risk of developing epilepsy increases with each passing decade.
The incidence of a first seizure is 52–59 per 100,000 in persons 40–59
years of age, but rise to 127 per 100,000 in those 60 and over. Among persons 65 years and older, the active epilepsy prevalence rate (the percent of
the total population who have a disorder) is approximately 1.5%, which
is about twice the rate of younger adults. As the elderly population continues to grow more people are likely to develop epilepsy and receive

Table 7-1   Proposed Division of Elderly

65–74 years	75–84 years	85 years and older
Young-old, healthy	Middle-old, healthy	Oldest-old, healthy
Young-old, multiple medical problems	Middle-old, multiple medical problems	Oldest-old, multiple medical problems
Young-old, frail	Middle-old, frail	Oldest-old, frail

AEDs. The causes of epilepsy in the elderly differ from those in younger adults. The most common identifiable cause of epilepsy is stroke, which accounts for 30%–40% of all cases where the cause is known. Brain tumor, head injury, and Alzheimer's disease are other major causes. In approximately half of the cases, the precise cause cannot be identified and are diagnosed as cryptogenic in the elderly. A major problem, however, is that many seizures may not be epileptic, that is, originating within the brain. Convulsive syncope (Chapter 1), provoked by a lack of circulation to the brain, is of particular concern. This is not epilepsy and the treatment must be directed towards the cardiac cause. While most elderly have complex partial seizures, there are difficulties encountered in making an accurate diagnosis because physicians usually think only of convulsions.

Many physicians begin treatment after a single convulsive seizure in older patients because the occurrence of a second seizure is high if a lesion in the central nervous system (e.g., tumor, stroke, AVM) is present. Also, the risk of serious injury is greater in the elderly. However, treatment in the older person carries more risks than in younger persons because the elderly may experience more side effects, have a greater risk for drug interactions, and be less able to afford the cost of medications.

Assessment of AED treatment results and toxicity in older patients is challenging because seizures are sometime difficult to observe. Signs and symptoms of toxicity can be attributed to other causes (e.g., Alzheimer's disease, stroke, etc.) or to co-medications and the elderly patients may not be able to accurately self-report problems. Extra attention to the evaluation of the elderly patients treated with AEDs is required.

In addition to their use in epilepsy, AEDs are prescribed for a variety of other disorders, including neuralgias (nerve pain), aggressive behavior, essential tremor, and restless legs syndrome—conditions prevalent in the elderly. Treatment of older patients with AEDs, as with many other medications, is complicated by increased sensitivity to drug effects, narrow therapeutic ranges, and the increased likelihood of drug interactions because of multiple drug therapy. As a cause of adverse reactions among the elderly, AEDs rank fifth among all drug categories.

Epilepsy and AED use is very common in nursing homes. A large nursing home database, which has information about the diagnosis of every nursing home resident over 65 years of age, shows that during 2001 approximately 10% of all nursing home residents were being treated with an AED. Approximately 7% had a diagnosis of epilepsy listed and the others were being treated with an AED for behavioral conditions or pain. Approximately 1.5 million elderly people reside in nursing homes; thus, as many as 150,000 nursing home elderly may be taking AEDs.

CLINICAL PHARMACOLOGY OF AEDS IN THE ELDERLY

The AED concentration in the brain determines both the antiseizure and the toxic effects of the drug. This is why measuring the levels of AEDs can be helpful in guiding treatment. The usual test for AED concentration measures the total concentration in the blood. But blood contains both drugs that are in the liquid part of the serum (unbound or free) and drug that is attached (bound) to proteins. Only the unbound drug concentration in serum is in direct equilibrium (balance) with the concentration at the site of action. Therefore, measurement of the unbound concentration is the best measure of activity.

However, measuring the unbound concentration requires an extra step and doubles the cost of the test, although it provides the best correlation with drug response. Most AEDs are not highly protein bound and measuring the total (free plus bound) is adequate. Two of the major AEDs (phenytoin and valproic acid) are highly bound, and binding is frequently altered in older persons. This is because they may be receiving other drugs that may change the binding, or they may have lower amounts of serum protein. In these patients, measuring the total concentration underestimates the actual amount of AED at the site of the action. A reading of the total level, which seems to be in the safe range, may actually be too high. To give an example, phenytoin is usually 90% bound and 10% free. This means that if the total level is measured at 20mg/L, the free or unbound is 2mg/L. Most younger adults have an effective range of 10–20 mg/L total, which means the effective range for free or unbound is 1–2 mg/L.

Many elderly, however, may have only 80% bound and 20% free. This means that if a total in an older person is 20 mg/L, the free is actually 4 mg/L (20% of 20). An older person with a free level this high may appear to have Alzheimer's or Parkinson's disease—acting confused, shaky, and unable to walk. A physician who does not know about free levels may see a total level of 20 mg/L (acceptable for a younger person) and not realize that the problems are caused by too much phenytoin. Lowering the level of phenytoin may reverse most of the problems with confusion and walking. Unfortunately, the concentration values used to guide treatment in younger persons for phenytoin, valproate and carbazepine may be too high for older persons. Unbound or free levels should be measured in elderly if they are receiving a highly protein bound drug.

It has generally been assumed that as one ages, metabolism slows down. Some studies involving small numbers of older persons seemed to show this, but more recent studies are giving a more complicated picture. There are two major systems in the liver. The first involves a group of enzymes made up of the cytochrome p-450 oxidative system. This is the largest system and metabolizes carbamazepine, phenytoin, valproate, Phenobarbital, felbamate, topiramate, oxcarbazepine, and zonisamide. Newer studies are showing that while this system does slow down with age, the amount it slows is different for each person. Some healthy people in their 90s metabolize phenytoin almost as rapidly as some younger adults, and some people in their 60s have a much slower metabolism. Some of this may be related to the health and lifestyle they may have had when they were younger. Consequently, a blanket statement that everyone's liver slows down with age cannot be made. Each person needs to be evaluated individually and doses determined accordingly.

The glucuronidation system is the other major metabolizing system in the liver. Lamotrigine is the AED that is principally metabolized by

118

this system, although other AEDs have some of their metabolism by this enzyme also. Very few studies have been done in drugs that use this system, but the little that is known would seem to show that glucuronidation is little affected by age. However, this system is greatly affected by estrogen, and it is not know how much the glucuronidation system is affected by menopause and hormone replacement therapy.

The other major route for elimination of drugs is through the urine. Gabapentin, levetiracetam, and pregabalin are eliminated almost exclusively by the kidney. Unlike the progress of liver function with age, kidney (renal) function has been well studied, and there appears to be a steady decrease in function of approximately 10% each decade. Doses of these drugs definitely need to be reduced as the years go by. Again, however, not every person has the same degree of change, so measuring levels of AEDs periodically would be helpful.

AEDs Commonly Used in Older Persons

Phenytoin

The AED phenytoin has been available since 1938 and is still the most widely used AED by the elderly. It makes up 50%–60% of all AED use by community dwelling and nursing home elderly. However, it has a narrow therapeutic range and complex pharmokinetics. It is absorbed slowly and is approximately 90% bound to serum albumin.

Smaller maintenance doses of phenytoin are needed in the elderly to attain desired unbound serum concentrations, and relatively small changes in does (less than 10%) are recommended when making dosing adjustments. In the elderly, a daily does of 3 mg/kg appears to be appropriate, rather than the 5 mg/kg per day used in younger adults. This 3 mg/kg dose is only 160 mg/day for a 52-kg (115 pound) woman, or 200 mg/day for a 66-kg (145 pound) man.

One nursing home survey revealed that residents were taking phenytoin doses similar to those used in younger adults. Consequently, there is a great potential for inadvertent overdose in the nursing home population. A range of 5 mg/L to 10 mg/L total, rather than the 10-20 mg/L used for younger persons may be more appropriate as a therapeutic range for the elderly.

Valproic Acid

Valproic acid (valproate) appears to be the second most commonly used AED in nursing homes. It is often used for control of behavior as well as epilepsy. Valproic acid, like phenytoin, is associated with reduced protein binding and unbound clearance in the elderly. As a result, the desired clinical response may be achieved with a lower dose than usual. Because the serum elimination half-life is prolonged, the dosing interval can be extended. If the albumin concentration has fallen or the patient's clinical response does not correlate with total drug concentration, measurement of unbound drug should be considered.

Carbamazepine

Carbamazepine is used almost as much as valproate in the elderly. A few studies have shown that its elimination may be more affected by age than phenytoin, but more studies are needed. As for the other drugs, usually lower doses need to be used. Carbamazepine also has a tendency to lower sodium levels and should not be used with diuretics, which also have this effect.

DRUG INTERACTIONS

Other medications taken by elderly patients can alter the absorption, distribution, and metabolism of AEDs, thereby increasing the risk of toxicity or therapeutic failure. For example, calcium-containing antacids and sucralfate reduce the absorption of phenytoin. The absorption of phenytoin, carbamazepine, and valproate may be reduced significantly by oral antineoplastic drugs (drugs used to treat cancer) that damage gastrointestinal cells. In addition, phenytoin concentrations may be lowered by intravenously administered antineoplastic agents. The use of folic acid for the treatment of megaloblastic anemia may decrease serum concentrations of phenytoin, and enteral (nasogastric tube)feeding can also lower serum concentrations in patients receiving orally administered phenytoin.

Many drugs displace AEDs from plasma proteins, an effect that is especially serious when the interacting drug also inhibits the metabolism of the displaced drug. This occurs when valproate interacts with phenytoin. Several drugs used on a short-term basis (including propoxyphene and erythromycin) or as maintenance therapy (such as cimetidine, diltiazem, fluoxetine, and verapamil) significantly inhibit the metabolism of one or more AEDs by the P-450 system. Certain agents can induce (i.e., speed up) the P-450 system or other enzymes, causing an increase in drug metabolism. The most commonly prescribed inducers of drug metabolism are phenytoin, phenobarbital, and carbamazepine. Ethanol (alcohol), when used chronically, also induces drug metabolism.

The interaction between antipsychotic drugs and AEDs is complex. Hepatic metabolism of certain antipsychotics such as haloperidol can be increased by carbamazepine, resulting in diminished psychotropic response. Antipsychotic medications, especially chlorpromazine, promazine, trifluoperazine, and perphenazine, can reduce the threshold for seizures. The risk of seizures is directly proportional to the total number of psychotropic medications being taken, their doses, any abrupt increases in doses, and the presence of organized brain pathology. The patient with epilepsy taking antipsychotic drugs may need a higher dose of antiepileptic mediation to control seizures. In contrast, central nervous system depressants are likely to lower the maximum dose of AEDs that can be administered before toxic symptoms occur.

In summary, treating epilepsy in the elderly is very complicated. One must carefully identify the cause of seizures (epileptic or nonepileptic). Use of AEDs is difficult because of possible side-effects, overmedication, drug interactions, and other issues.

CHAPTER 8

Epilepsy and Quality of Life

M OST PEOPLE WITH EPILEPSY can live near-normal lives. While there are certain limits on occupations, such as aircraft pilot and commercial vehicle driver, most lifestyles are possible. Unnecessary barriers are due often to misunderstandings. In the United States, the Americans with Disabilities Act has been very beneficial in allowing persons with epilepsy to get and keep jobs. Participation in sports, education, families, and other activities are all possible.

SPORTS

Participation in sports is important. This is particularly the case for young persons in school, where being on a team can be a major learning experience. Unfortunately, many parents and school officials use the excuse of preventing injury to unnecessarily limit epileptic students' participation in sports. This need not be the case (Table 8-1). A number of successful athletes have epilepsy. One example is a member of the USA 2006 Olympic hockey team who is an Epilepsy Foundation advocate for persons with epilepsy participating in sports. There is little or no evidence that physical fatigue such as that experienced in strenuous activity will lead to a seizure. Indeed, one person with epilepsy runs marathon races and has never had a seizure while running but may have a seizure a few days after a race.

Common sense should be used in choosing sporting activities. In general, activities that involve the possibility of significant metabolic imbalances, such as scuba diving or high-altitude mountain climbing, should be avoided. Also, sports that involve the potential for serious injury from

Table 8-1   Sports/Activities and Epilepsy

Permitted Sports/Activities—No Restrictions

Aerobics	Dancing	Lacrosse
Archery	Dog sledding	Orienteering
Badminton	Discus throwing	Running
Ballet	Fencing	Shot putting
Baseball	Field hockey	Skiing—cross country
Basketball	High jumping	Soccer
Bowling	Fishing	Softball
Broad jumping	Gymnastics	Table tennis
Cricket	Golf	Volleyball
Croquet	Hiking	Weightlifting
Curling	Jogging	Wrestling

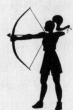

Possible Sports/Activities—Reasonable Precautions

Bicycling	Ice skating	Skating
Bobsledding	Karate	Skiing—downhill
Canoeing	Kayaking	Sledding
Diving	Mountain climbing	Snorkeling
Football	Pole vaulting	Snowmobiling
Horseback riding	Rollerblading	Swimming
Hockey	Rugby	Tennis
Hunting	Sailing	Water polo

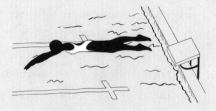

Prohibited Sports/Activities

Boxing	Polo	Skydiving
Bungee jumping	Rock climbing	Surfing
Hang gliding	Sail boarding	Waterskiing
Jousting	Scuba diving	

loss of consciousness should be avoided. These include sports in which the body does not have contact with the ground, such as skydiving.

Also, sports that carry a high risk for head injury should be avoided. Location and surroundings also play a role. Swimming, if done in a well-lighted pool with lifeguard or others aware of the swimmer's epilepsy, is possible. On the other hand, swimming in a river or lake should be avoided. Some years ago, the American Medical Association's Committee on Medical Aspects of Sports published the following statement: "There is ample evidence that patients with epilepsy will not be affected by indulging in any sport, including football, provided the normal safeguards for sports participation are followed, including adequate head projection." However, boxing is prohibited because it is well-known to be associated with repeated head injury, even with protective gear.

EMPLOYMENT

With the exception of certain occupations, a person with epilepsy should be able to work at any job for which they have the ability. Seizures in most cases happen relatively rarely at the workplace. If co-workers are educated about first aid (see Chapter 1) and understand that persons usually recover quickly after a seizure, the workplace can be a satisfactory experience for all. Often, employers are reluctant to hire someone with epilepsy because of worries about liability if an injury happens on the job or simply a misunderstanding of the condition. Although the Epilepsy Foundation has been working to educate the public about epilepsy, a great deal of misunderstanding still exists. In many cases, however, the person with epilepsy is often a very loyal and hardworking employee because they are aware of the difficulties of finding a job. In many cases, once an employer is comfortable with hiring a person with epilepsy, they are very pleased with the work performance. Overall, a person with epilepsy's attitude, work habits and ability to work with others is more important to having a positive work experience than the fact that they have occasional seizures.

Today, there are only a few job categories which are closed to the person with epilepsy. These are ones which involve public safety. For example, piloting an aircraft, driving a large truck, being in a combat zone, or working as an emergency service provider. On the other hand, because of improved safety standards now required to protect all workers, many jobs previously off-limits now may be possible. These include working in high places because all workers in these jobs must now wear safety harnesses and have other protections such as guard rails. Machinery now must have special switches which turn the equipment off in case the worker looses consciousness or control.

Sometimes the condition which caused the epilepsy may also be associated with limits in the brain's ability to work normally. The most common problem faced by many persons with epilepsy is memory loss. This is because the temporal lobes are the structures which process memory, and are also the areas of the brain most likely to be the source of complex partial seizures. The right temporal lobe usually processes memory for pictures and maps (visual memory). The left temporal lobe processes memory for speech (verbal memory). In many cases, only one temporal lobe is not working normally. With special testing (psychometric testing) one can measure the degree to which these different types of memory are affected. This can be of great help in career decisions and helping develop the best learning strategies. For example, if a person has very poor visual memory but excellent verbal memory, careers such as architecture, engineering or other occupations which require the ability to remember structures and relationships between objects would not be good choices. On the other hand, jobs remembering what people said would be good work choices. Also, if it is discovered early enough, children with verbal memory problems should be in teaching settings where pictures are used more.

GETTING HELP WITH WORK OR DISABILITY

The Americans With Disabilities Act, passed in 1990, specifically includes persons with epilepsy. The Act is intended to prevent discrimination at the workplace. This starts by having regulations against the employer from asking about disabilities during the hiring process, and focusing only on the abilities. Once a person is hired, appropriate accommodations must then be provided. For persons with epilepsy who have no limitations other than an occasional seizure, very little needs to be done in the way of accommodations. There are however many different interpretations about each specific situation so sometimes help is needed in settling disputes.

Social Security benefits are available to persons whose epilepsy is severe enough to make it impossible to get competitive employment. To get help, the first step is for a physician to certify the presence of epilepsy which has not been controlled. Although the applications of the regulations vary somewhat among the disability examiner, the usual criteria is that a person have at least one seizure which involves loss of consciousness or control each month in spite of adequate medical treatment. This would include complex partial seizures but not simple partial seizures. If the person does not have that many seizures but has other disabilities, these may also be taken into account. For example, fewer seizures but significant memory loss may also qualify. Usually disability is not granted for lifetime, rather it is re-evaluated periodically. Persons who are cured of their epilepsy by surgery may loose their disability status. Therefore, it is important that as a person's seizures are better controlled, help is obtained in making adjustments. The appendix lists some useful websites for additional information.

CHAPTER 9

Staying Healthy
with Epilepsy

TREATING COMMON ILLNESSES

EVERYONE DEVELOPS MEDICAL PROBLEMS ranging from common colds to more serious illnesses. Many of these are helped by various treatments including over-the-counter (OTC) and prescription medications. Although pharmacists today have long lists of warnings for prescription medicines, these may not always be appropriate for persons with epilepsy because they are overly detailed and the warnings are overstated so that otherwise useful medicines may be avoided. Table 9-1 gives a list of the most common problems a person with epilepsy may develop, along with some appropriate prescription and nonprescription treatments.

There are two general types of problems. The first is taking products that may stimulate or excite the brain, making it more likely to have a seizure. The other is using substances that interfere with the AEDs, either by increasing or decreasing their levels.

PERSONAL SAFETY

Injury during or after a seizure is a major concern, but there are many things that can be done to minimize injury. Perhaps the most important step that can be taken is to educate families, friends, and coworkers on what to do in case of a seizure. Most people do not know what to do and may panic or apply inappropriate first-aid measures.

Persons with localization-related epilepsy may have a simple partial seizure (aura) which permits precautions to be taken. Simple partial

Table 9-1 List of Medications That Should Be Avoided and Others That May Be Used If a Person Has Epilepsy and Needs to Be Treated for Common Conditions

Category	Avoid use	Safe to use	Discuss with your physician
Antibiotics/antifungals	If on Tegretol: Biaxin (clarithromycin) Erythromycin Pediazole (Erythoagen and sulfisoxazole)	Zithromax (azithromycin)	Diflucan (fluconazole) Sporanox (itraconazole) Doxycycline, Bio-Tab, Doxy, Vibramycin Flagyl (metronidazole)
Blood thinner			Aspirin (ED ASA) or Coumadin (warfarin)
Constipation and diarrhea		Imodium AD (loperamide) Colace (docusate sodium) Metamucil (psylium) Dulcolaz (bisacodyl)	
Cough/cold/allergy remedies	Cold products containing alcohol Cold or allergy products containing phenylephrine or phenylpropanolamine (Contact, Dimetapp, Tavist-D) Astemizole (hismanal)	Dimetane (brompheramine) Chloraseptic (benzocaine) Sore throat lozenges (any type) Chlor-Trimeton (chlorpheneramine) Cold products containing dextromethorphan (Robitussin DM) Cold products containing guiafenesin (Robitussin) Polaramine (dexchlorpheniramine) Sudafed (pseudoephedrine) Allegra (fexofenadine) Zyrtec (cetirizine)	Benadryl (diphenhydramine) Claritin (loratidine)

(continued on next page)

Table 9-1 List of Medications That Should Be Avoided and Others That May Be Used If a Person Has Epilepsy and Needs to Be Treated for Common Conditions (continued)

Category	Avoid use	Safe to use	Discuss with your physician
Heartburn and stomach upset	Tagamet (cimetidine)	Zantac (ranitidine) Pepcid (famotidine) Axid (nizatidine) Mylanta, Maalox, Gaviscon—space 2 hrs. from antiepileptic medications	Prilosec (omeprazole) Carafate (sucralfate)
Herbal products	St. Johns Wort Metabolife 356		Ginkobeloba Echinecea
Hormone replacement and birth control			Hormonal contraceptives: birth control pills, Depo Provera, Norplant Premarin and other hormonal replacement therapy
Mental health			Wellbutrin (bupropion) Prozac (fluoxetine) Zoloft Lithium
Pain and fever	Darvon, Darvocet-Propoxyphene If on Felbatol: Tylenol (acetaminophen)	Advil, Motrin, Ketoprofen (Orudis), generic ibuprofen or other NSAIDs for short periods Vicodin Tylenol #3 If not on Felbatol: Tylenol (acetaminophen) for short periods	Ibuprofen or other NSAIDs in high doses

(continued on next page)

131

Table 9-1 List of Medications That Should Be Avoided and Others That May Be Used If a Person Has Epilepsy and Needs to Be Treated for Common Conditions (continued)

Category	Avoid use	Safe to use	Discuss with your physician
Smoking cessation aids		Nicoderm Patch Nicoderm Gum	Zyban (bupropion)
Vitamin supplements		Mutivitamin with minerals and folic acid and without caffeine (Vitamin A-Z) Calcium supplement–space 2 hrs from antiepileptic medications)	
Other	Alcohol Street drugs of any kind Avoid another person's prescription drugs		Generic antiepileptic drugs Theophylline (Aerolate, Siobid, Theo-dur) Antabuse (disulfiram) Isoniazid

Developed by MINCEP® Epilepsy Care. Copyright © 1997. Revised 2001. Used by permission. Minnesota Comprehensive Epilepsy Program (MINCEP®) is a trademark and licensed to MINCEP® Epilepsy Care.

seizures may be a jerking of a muscle group, a feeling in a part of the body, a sensation in the stomach (similar to the downward part of a roller coaster ride), flashing light, or a *deja vu* sensation. Some persons have learned that by some action (such as grabbing an arm or intense focused mental concentration), they may stop the seizure. In one case, a woman with an olfactory (strong smell) aura could block a seizure by smelling a perfume container. However, many people have not found a way to block a secondary generalized tonic-clonic seizure, and they must take action to prevent injury. This should include sitting or, preferably, lying down, removing any objects from the mouth that could cause choking, and moving away from furniture with sharp corners.

Persons who have complex partial seizures that proceed to generalized tonic-clonic seizures may not be able to protect themselves. During the complex partial seizure, the person may wander aimlessly, open and close doors, unbutton or unzip clothes, or touch others persons inappropriately. Rarely is there aggressive behavior; and, if it happens, it is often not premeditated or appropriate. Rather, it may be a response to attempts at restraint or loud instructions that are not comprehended. Aid should consist of gentle guiding away from harmful objects. Perhaps most important is reassuring other people that this is a medical condition (not intentional socially unacceptable behavior or criminal activity) and that it will cease in a few minutes. If the person starts having jerking (clonic activity), she or he should be guided to a sitting or lying position.

The seizures most likely to cause injury are generalized tonic-clonic seizures. Generalized tonic-clonic seizures consist of complete loss of consciousness, stiffening of all body muscles, and falling, either backward or forward, hitting the front or back of the head. Then there is very strong jerking of the arms and legs. Trying to hold a person still during a convulsion may cause injury to both you and the person.

When the seizure is over in two or three minutes, there is very heavy breathing and a gradual return of consciousness. Because the body is starved for oxygen after a seizure, breathing must not be blocked. The tongue may be bitten during a seizure, and it has become common practice to try to force something into the mouth of a person having a convulsion. This approach has been shown in films (*Cleopatra,*

1963, in which Julius Caesar is shown having a round stick forced between his teeth) and in almost all first aid books written before 1980. Research has shown that trying to force something into the mouth may break teeth, cause vomiting, and block breathing. In the past, padded tongue blades were kept at bedsides in hospitals, but these have now been removed.

Also, the jerking movements should not be restrained. They are often so strong that attempts to hold arms or legs in place causes injury. Rather, harmful objects in the vicinity should be removed. After the seizure, the persons should be turned to one side so that any saliva or blood can drain and so the tongue is not falling back into the throat, which may block breathing. If a person is known to have epilepsy and does not injure him- or herself during a seizure, 911 does not need to be called. Most persons will recover within 10–15 minutes. One of the major complaints people with epilepsy have is that too often an ambulance is called, and they are taken to a hospital. By the time they get to the hospital, they have recovered but are often left with an expensive bill to pay.

BRACELETS, NECKLACES, AND CARDS

Various bracelets and necklaces are available to identify persons with various medical conditions (Figure 9-1). People with frequent seizures should have one to identify who they are and what their medical condition is and to provide contact information for relatives or friends. It is also essential that a list of all medicines and doses, as well as a list of

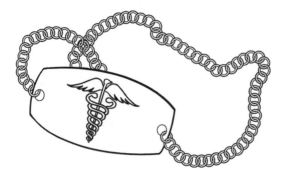

FIGURE 9-1

Medical bracelet.

allergies, be carried by the person in a wallet or purse so that in case of emergency the proper treatment can be given in an emergency.

DIET

In general, persons with epilepsy do not need special diets. A well-balanced diet with fruits and vegetables is appropriate. Because some AEDs speed up metabolism of some vitamins, a once-a day multivitamin is appropriate. Excessive amounts of vitamins need not be given. A general rule is to avoid excesses. Caffeine in large quantities can cause seizures, so generally avoiding more than 5 cups of regular coffee is recommended. Similarly, many beverages contain excessive caffeine. A general principle is to avoid any which promise extra energy or wakefulness.

There are some rare forms of epilepsy which may be helped by diet. Some infants have seizures which can be only controlled by vitamin B_6 (pyridoxine). Some adults may have seizures associated with magnesium deficiency. Consequently, some non-medical magazines or promoters of non-tested remedies tout the virtues of various substances such as B vitamins in high doses, mineral supplements, taurine and other substances which may have some remote association with medical literature but have not been proven to be of value to most persons with epilepsy. Unfortunately most of these "remedies" are costly and may drain resources from families already facing many expenses. Also, there is no evidence that adults with epilepsy are helped by B_6 and actually, high doses of B_6 have been reported to cause nerve damage.

The most useful diet for epilepsy is the ketogenic diet. It was developed in the early 1920's when only bromide and phenobarbital were available. Many studies were done using this diet, but it fell out of general use after it was shown that phenytoin, introduced in 1938, was much more effective for most adults and children. However, there are a few children with very severe epilepsy for whom this diet is very effective and appropriate. With the ketogenic diet, almost all of the calories are replaced by fats, with very little protein and no carbohydrates. Even one piece of candy can eliminate the effects of the diet. The theory of the diet is that if the body gets only fat, the whole metabolism changes and makes the bran less likely to have seizures. It is started in the hospital and for the first few days the person experiences weakness, nausea and other symptoms. These usually clear. The diet requires constant attention to preparing meals which can be acceptable. Interestingly, most children on this diet loose weight and become thin. Also, there may be some long term effects.On the other hand, for the children for whom this diet is appropriate, the seizure control achieved may outweigh the negative effects. Because the Atkins diet is also a high fat diet, there has been some speculation that it may be beneficial for adults with epilepsy. However, no large-scale study has been done to prove this.

WEIGHT CONTROL AND DIETING

Weight control is a problem for many persons, but may be especially problematic for some persons with epilepsy. This is because some do not get enough exercise because of unnecessary limits. Others are being treated with AEDs which are associated with weight gain. While most persons taking valproate, gabapentin or pregabalin do not gain a significant amount of, weight, some do. On the other hand, felbamate, topiramate and zonisamide are associated with weight loss.

Unfortunately many drugs and natural products which are marketed for weight loss can cause seizures in persons who do not have epilepsy and make seizures worse in persons who have this disorder. This is because products which claim to produce weight loss by "speeding up" metabolism are strong stimulants of the brain and cause seizures by making it over excitable. Many of these products also increase blood pressure. The only safe way to increase metabolism is by using muscles. Persons with epilepsy or afraid of having a seizure should avoid any product which promises to provide an easy way to lose weight.

SLEEP

Getting enough sleep is important. Physicians often use sleep deprivation before an EEG to increase the chance of recording epileptiform activity. Many persons with epilepsy report more seizures after missing sleep. Many young persons who stay up late on weekends have provoked seizures. Persons with epilepsy should not have employment requiring shift changes. For example, nurses with epilepsy can work the night shift consistently, but should not be frequently switched from the night to the day shift.

The amount of sleep one needs differs between persons. The average is 8 hours, but some do well on only 5 or 6, while others need 10 hours or more. The best way to know if you have had enough sleep is to see how you get through the day. It is normal to feel a little tired in the middle of the morning, feel sleepy after lunch, and nod off in a darkened room with a boring lecture. However, nodding off while driving, being with someone interesting, or walking are signs of sleep deprivation. Some persons with epilepsy have mostly nighttime seizures and lose sleep because of these. Sometimes using a short acting anti-seizure medicine such as lorazepam which also is a sleep-inducer can be helpful. Some persons with epilepsy also have sleep-apnea. A continuous 24 hour EEG done by epilepsy centers can often sort out sleep problems.

STRESS

Studies have shown that emotional stress can make seizures worse in a person with epilepsy. Interestingly, the study showed that good news stress was just as likely to cause seizures as bad news stress. This is probably because excitement of any kind modifies the delicate balance of the brain. Stress is unavoidable in life, so the best approach is to learn how to deal with stress. Sometimes this can be helped by counseling. If there are constant stressors present, one should try to eliminate these by altering work or relationship issues.

However, stress will not cause epileptic seizures in a person who does not have epilepsy. Many persons with stress have non-epileptic psychogenic seizures (see Chapter 1). These must be accurately diagnosed to avoid inappropriate use of AEDs and causing problems with driving and work.

DEPRESSION

In broad terms, there are two types of depression: situational and endogenous. Situational depressions develop after a major negative event in life such as the death of a loved one or onset of a major medical illness. Endogenpous depression may be independent of life-events and is thought to be a disturbance of brain chemistry. Depression is common among persons with epilepsy and they may have one or both types of depression. Often situational depression develops after seizures start. Loss of driving privileges, changes in relationships and issues at work often contribute to this. Usually this type of depression improves with readjustments in life style, better understanding of the disorder, and support and understanding from close ones. Endogenous depression can often be improved by use of medicines used to treat depression. A very clear diagnosis of the type of depression needs to be made to get the most effective treatment. Sometimes the lack of drive and a negative outlook caused by depression is more debilitating than a few seizures. The quality of life can often be improved as much or more by treating depression than by decreasing seizures. Focusing just on seizure control without also recognizing the disruptive role of depression will not lead to the best outcome.

CHAPTER 10

Driving
and Seizures

EVERY STATE REGULATES driver license eligibility. This often includes specific standards for persons with medical conditions. Each state has its own regulations regarding driving and epilepsy. Table 10-1 gives a summary of the key points. These regulations are of course subject to change. The area of greatest change in the last few years has been the seizure-free period. In the past, most states required a one-year period from the time of the last seizure. But because of increasing recognition that people with epilepsy do not differ significantly in overall driving safety from the general population, many states are liberalizing the requirements by shortening the time from the last seizure to restitution of driving privileges. Some states have removed the terms "seizure" and "epilepsy" from their statutes and refer instead to episodes of loss of consciousness, loss of control, and/or loss of awareness. This includes by implication conditions other than epilepsy (such as diabetes, heart disease) in their regulations. Some states also have medical review boards that will grant exceptions to the general rules. Some of these exceptions may include the following:

- a breakthrough seizure caused by a physician-directed change in medications;
- an isolated seizure wherein medical examination indicates that another seizure appears unlikely;
- a seizure related to a temporary illness;
- an established pattern of only nocturnal seizures;
- an established pattern of seizures that does not impair driving ability; that is, simple partial seizures with no loss of consciousness or control.

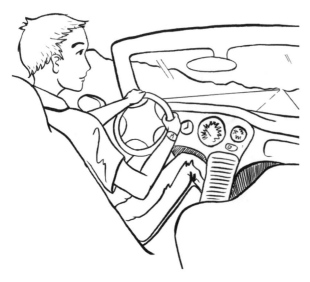

FIGURE 10-1

Driving safely is possible for many persons with epilepsy with proper treatment.

One area of uncertainty is the action to be taken after a single seizure. Should a person have his or her driving restricted after a single seizure? This question does not have a simple answer. One must balance the small probability of a second seizure occurring while driving against the considerable loss of income, freedom, and self-esteem experienced by someone losing a driver's license.

In most states, the person with epilepsy has the responsibility to report to the state the development of epilepsy or the occurrence of a seizure. In these states, the physician must counsel patients on their responsibilities and document on the medical record that this has been done. This preserves the confidentiality of the physician–patient relationship, and patients can freely discuss their condition with their physicians.

Unfortunately, six states—California, Delaware, Nevada, New Jersey, Oregon, and Pennsylvania—have mandatory physician-reporting requirements. While the exact terms of these provisions vary, they generally require any physician who diagnoses or treats a patient with epilepsy to report that patient's name, age, and address to a state agency, usually the Department of Motor Vehicles or the Department of Public Safety.

Most physicians feel that mandatory reporting laws are counterproductive because they erode the confidential nature of the physician–patient relationship. Proper diagnosis and treatment of

Table 10-1 State Regulations for Driving

State	Seizure-Free Period
Alabama	6 months, with exceptions
Alaska	6 months
Arizona	3 months, with exceptions
Arkansas	1 year
California	3, 6, or 12 months, with exceptions
Colorado	No set seizure-free period
Connecticut	No set seizure-free period
Delaware	No set seizure-free period
District of Columbia	1 year
Florida	Upon doctor's recommendation
Georgia	6 months
Hawaii	6 months, with exceptions
Idaho	6 months, with strong recommendation from doctor
Illinois	No set seizure-free period
Indiana	No set seizure-free period
Iowa	6 months; less if seizures nocturnal
Kansas	6 months; less if seizures nocturnal
Kentucky	90 days
Louisiana	6 months, with doctor's statement
Maine	3 months or longer
Maryland	No set seizure-free period
Massachusetts	6 months; less with doctor's statement
Michigan	6 months; less at discretion of department
Minnesota	6 months, with exceptions
Mississippi**	1 year
Missouri**	6 months, with doctor's recommendation
Montana++	No set seizure-free period; doctor's recommendation
Nebraska++	3 months
Nevada	3 months, with exceptions
New Hampshire++	1 year; less at discretion of department
New Jersey	1 year; less on recommendation of committee
New Mexico	1 year, less on recommendation of advisory board
New York	1 year, with exceptions

(continued on next page)

Table 10-1   State Regulations for Driving (continued)

State	Seizure-Free Period
North Carolina	6-12 months, with exceptions
North Dakota	6 months; restricted license possible after 3 months
Ohio	No set seizure-free period
Oklahoma	6 months
Oregon	6 months, with exceptions
Pennsylvania	6 months, with exceptions
Puerto Rico	No set seizure-free period
Rhode Island	18 months; less at discretion of department
South Carolina	6 months
South Dakota	6-12 months, less with doctor's recommendation
Tennessee	6 months, with acceptable medical form
Texas	6 months, with doctor's recommendation
Utah	3 months
Vermont	No set seizure-free period
Virginia	6 months, with exceptions
Washington	6 months, with exceptions
West Virginia	1 year, with exceptions
Wisconsin	3 months, with acceptable medical form
Wyoming	3 months

BOLD = mandatory physician reporting
** = no appeal of denial of license
++ = no periodic medical updates required
Modified from Epilepsy Foundation of America information. Copyright Epilepsy Foundation. All rights reserved. Reprinted with permission.

epilepsy depend greatly on the development of an honest, trusting relationship between a patient and the physician. Accurate information concerning seizure activity is critically important. If patients know or fear that their doctors are obligated to report their seizures to the state, they may withhold crucial information to avoid state sanctions. That nondisclosure of essential information could result in inadequate treatment and more seizures.

At the federal level, the U.S. Department of Transportation has regulations that bar anyone with any history of seizures or epilepsy from being licensed to drive in interstate trucking. Again, however, individual exceptions may be made where there is evidence that the epilepsy has been cured.

Tort law in many states has recognized that physicians may be held liable for damages arising from the acts of their patients. Because of this concern regarding lawsuits, physicians must strictly apply the laws which exist in their states.

The Epilepsy Foundation maintains an online resource concerning state driving laws http://www.epilepsyfoundation.org/answerplace/Social/driving/.

Be sure to check with the proper government office in your own state for the latest rules.

CHAPTER 11

Stopping AEDS and Status Epilepticus

FOR MANY PEOPLE WITH EPILEPSY, treatment does not need to be life-long. Children with certain epileptic syndromes such as childhood absence epilepsy or benign rolandic epilepsy can stop medications by the early teenage years or sooner. Many adults may also be able to stop medications, but this has to be done carefully.

In general, if the epilepsy has been caused by a severe head injury, brain tumor, encephalitis, malformation of the brain, or other severe structural causes, it is unlikely that medications should be stopped even if seizures have been fully controlled for many years. Persons for whom medication discontinuation is most likely to succeed are those who have cryptogenic (i.e., no know cause) epilepsy, who had control of seizures quickly after treatment was started, who have normal EEGs, who have had normal MRI scans and are not having "auras," that is, small simple partial seizures. Even then, a study that followed persons taken off medicines for 10 years found that approximately 1 out of 10 had another seizure.

Persons who have had mesial temporal sclerosis and for whom surgery has been successful are also candidates for discontinuation of AEDs. The primary goal of temporal lobectomy is the elimination of seizures. Discontinuation of medicines is a secondary goal. In most cases, physicians will try to reduce some medicines a few months after surgery, and after one year reduce the level to just one. That one may be continued up to four years after surgery, and then, if the EEG is favorable and there have been no auras, AEDs can be discontinued gradually. Some patients who have had very frequent seizures for many years before surgery and are having no side effects from the medicine are reluctant to discontinue AEDs. Physicians should not force patients to discontinue AEDs

145

against their will. The decision to stop medication must be made by a physician who is familiar with the risks and benefits of withdrawing AEDs, and the person discontinuing the AED should be aware of the small risk of having seizures in the future.

STATUS EPILEPTICUS

AEDs should never be stopped abruptly but rather tapered off over a few months. Sudden stopping of AEDs may lead to status epilepticus. This is a life-threatening condition in which one generalized tonic-clonic seizure is followed by a second one within a few hours or less, before recovery from the first. Sometimes the seizures are almost continuous. Status epilepticus sometimes happens to persons who have never had seizures but suddenly begin to have very frequent generalized tonic-clonic seizures caused by a new problem in the brain such as bleeding, infection, or brain tumor. Sometimes it is caused by drug abuse. Status epilepticus is also common in persons with epilepsy who miss their medications.

Before the 1980s, as many as half of all persons with status epilepticus did not survive or suffered serious damage to the brain. Today, with much better treatments including intravenous benzodiazepams, fosphenytoin, valproate, and some newer drugs that will soon be available, the outlook is much better. The goal, however, is the prevention of status epilepticus. The most important factor is to develop foolproof methods for never missing medications. Pill boxes or other devices to assure that one never runs out of medicines are essential tools for preventing status. Persons who may have more than one place to stay, such as a weekend cabin or relative's home, should have a small supply of their medicines at those locations in case they forget to bring their pills. There are now also "rescue" medicines available. These are liquid forms of diazepam and lorazepam of which 1 or 2 ml can be dropped into the cheek pouch of the mouth during or shortly after a seizure. These are similar to medicines used intravenously in the emergency room; but because they can be given at home, they may prevent the need to call 911 or give a head start to seizure control. For children, a rectal syringe with a premeasured dose of diazepam is available.

CHAPTER 12

Complications
of Epilepsy

ARE PERSONS WITH EPILEPSY RETARDED?

THERE IS A COMMON MISCONCEPTION that persons with epilepsy have lower intelligence than average, or have mental retardation. Many studies have been done testing the IQs of people with epilepsy. These studies have shown that most persons with epilepsy have normal or even high levels of intelligence. Overall, there is no significant difference between those with epilepsy and the general population. The misperception that persons with epilepsy are mentally slow has probably developed because some persons with mental retardation also have severe epilepsy with frequent seizures even with medical treatment. The more serious the brain damage causing mental retardation is, the more likely that person is to have epilepsy. Complications during labor and delivery, such as low oxygen, low blood sugar, bleeding into the brain and other conditions, can cause brain damage. A few years later, many of these children develop seizures and have significant problems with learning and behavior. Often the seizures start first, and then it is noticed that they also have other problems. Unfortunately, the seizures and medicines are often blamed for all of the problems. There are unrealistic expectations that if only the medicines were stopped or that seizures were controlled, the child would be normal.

The type of epilepsy is the best predictor of intelligence in a person with epilepsy. In general, having primary generalized epilepsy does not alter brain functioning significantly. Thus, those with juvenile myoclonic epilepsy or absence epilepsy of childhood have normal intelligence overall.

People with localization cryptogenic epilepsy are usually able to learn and work without significant problems. However, those with localization-related epilepsy caused by a stroke, brain tumor, head injury or other condition will have difficulties with the functions that were damaged. AEDs, if used properly, usually add little to the problems of learning, behavior and memory. But treatment must be done carefully in these patients because overmedication can often worsen the learning problems and behavior. If these develop during treatment, it is useful to get a blood level to make sure that the person is not overmedicated. Sometimes it is not possible to get complete control of seizures without using too much medicine. It is important to develop a plan in which a balance is reached between the best possible seizure control and the fewest side effects. Although the goal of treatment is no seizures/no side effects, this is not possible in the severest cases. One then needs to carefully identify the most serious seizures, the ones associated with injury, and work to control or eliminate these. Smaller seizures, such as complex partial seizures lasting less than a minute, may then need to be tolerated. Most people with epilepsy are comfortable with a few seizures each year and no daily side effects instead of no seizures but daily side effects.

Another reason for the perception that people with epilepsy are mentally slow probably came from the fact that some of the older AEDs had serious side effects. Bromide, the first effective medicine for the control of seizures, causes fatigue, slow thinking, and learning problems. Phenobarbital had similar effects. Before 1938, these were the most widely used AEDs, and their use probably caused problems. The newer AEDs have fewer problems. Bromide is no longer used in humans, and in the United States phenobarbital is used less and less. However, because it is so inexpensive, phenobarbital is still the most widely used AED in the world.

DOES EPILEPSY CAUSE DEPRESSION?

As many as 20% to 40% of people with epilepsy also suffer from depression. Depression, like epilepsy, has many causes. In general, one can divide depression into those caused by circumstances external to the brain, such as life situations or use of drugs, and depression caused by a chemical imbalance in the brain. There seems to be a direct connection between endogenous depression (i.e., depression from a chemical imbalance) and epilepsy. Studies have shown that people with endogenous depression are more likely to develop cryptogenic epilepsy after the depression starts than those who do not have depression.

Many people who do not have endogenous depression become depressed after they are diagnosed with epilepsy. This is because life changes such as no driving, fear of having seizures, others being afraid, limitations at work, and other issues understandably make one depressed. Also, many AEDs, especially when they are first used, cause tiredness or somnolence (sleepiness).

For some, the depression is more limiting than the epilepsy. With depression, one lacks energy, is tired, may sleep too much, and find it difficult to get through the day. Often, use of antidepressant medicines can be helpful. Newer antidepressants usually do not worsen epilepsy, although some of them have a warning about this. Before treating depression, one must identify the causes. If the depression is caused by fear and anxiety about epilepsy, education and counseling may be very helpful. If phenobarbital is being used, changing to another AED is often helpful. Many people who stop having seizures after successful surgery for epilepsy find that their depression improves. Medicines for depression often take many weeks to begin to work, so they must be given time to take effect. Some of the AEDs also have antidepressant effects and are actually used in persons who do not have epilepsy. If a person with epilepsy also has depression, a physician may want to choose an AED that has antidepressant properties and avoid those that may worsen it.

CAN EPILEPSY CAUSE MEMORY LOSS?

Many persons with epilepsy are aware of memory loss. There are many reasons for this. The most severe problems with memory are in people with mesial temporal sclerosis. This epilepsy syndrome affects a region called the hippocampus, which is located in the middle of the temporal lobe. It is so named because it resembles a seahorse, or *hippocampus* in

Latin. This structure is very important for memory processing. In a right-handed person, the hippocampus on the left side of the brain is used for verbal memory and is close to the area used for speech. The right hippocampus is used mostly for visual memory. If one temporal lobe is damaged in childhood, the normal side can take over the work of the other. In this case, memory may be normal. The WADA test (intracarotid amytal test described in Chapter 5), during which one side of the brain is put to sleep for a short time, is used to find out if the damaged temporal lobe can be removed without changing memory function. However, if the temporal lobes are damaged later in life, memory problems can be severe, with the rest of the brain functions being normal.

Again, the epilepsy syndrome is the key factor in determining how much memory will be affected. People with primary generalized epilepsies usually have minimal trouble with memory. People with localization related symptomatic epilepsy, especially after head injury with damage to the temporal lobes, can have disabling problems with memory.

During a complex partial seizure, the memory circuits of the hippocampus are involved in the abnormal electrical activity. A major feature of these seizures is a lack of memory for the event. After a generalized tonic-clonic seizure, many patients have trouble with memory functioning for hours or days, but eventually recover.

Although AEDs are often blamed for memory problems, most of the newer AEDs used in usual doses have only minor or no effects on memory. Having seizures is usually the much greater factor, and having frequent or uncontrolled seizures can, over time, worsen memory functioning.

CAN SEIZURES CAUSE BRAIN DAMAGE?

In general, having a few seizures does not cause noticeable problems with how the brain works. Many famous persons who had only a few seizures during their lifetimes were able to have very productive careers. Julius Caesar, Alfred Nobel, and Fyodor Dostoevsky are but a few examples from history. However, in the case of adults, having one episode of status epilepticus (Chapter 11) has been shown to decrease the IQ by

150

approximately 10 points. Having 10 generalized tonic-clonic seizures over 10 years can also cause a similar lowering of the IQ. Children's brains seem to be more resistant to damage from seizures. In children, learning difficulties are usually a result of the brain damage that also has caused the epilepsy.

Seizures that cause falls can cause result in brain damage from physical injury or bleeding into the brain. People with atonic seizures that cause falls or individuals with partial complex seizures who wander and fall are at the greatest risk.

CAN I DIE FROM A SEIZURE?

In one survey, dying during a seizure was listed as the major worry by over two-thirds of people with epilepsy. It is also a common worry for those close to the person with epilepsy. In reality, it is very unusual for a person to die during a seizure. Many studies have been done to determine the cause of death in persons with epilepsy. In general, persons with cryptogenic epilepsy and primary generalized epilepsy have normal life spans.

The highest risk of dying during seizures is during status epilepticus. Approximately one-half of elderly people who develop status epilepticus die either during the seizure or from its complications. This is because repeated seizures place a great strain on the heart, or because the condition leading to status, such as a stroke, also has a high mortality rate. In younger adults and children, the rate is lower but may still be from 10% to 30%, even with the appropriate emergency treatment. Before 1970, the death rate was much higher because treatment was not as effective. Today, with use of benzodiazepams and fosphenytoin, the death rate from just the seizures is much lower, and death is from the condition that caused status epilepticus. Anybody who has one generalized tonic-clonic seizure lasting more than 5 minutes and is not recovering consciousness should receive emergency treatment. Also, anybody having two or more generalized tonic-clonic seizures within a few hours needs to be taken to a medical facility.

Death from drowning during a seizure is most likely if a person is swimming in a lake or river. Swimming in supervised pools is much less dangerous. Fatal automobile accidents are very uncommon in people whose epilepsy is controlled well enough to allow them to have a valid driver's license. Death from accidental injury during a seizure is also uncommon.

The most common cause of death, other than status epilepticus, in people with epilepsy is a condition known as sudden unexpected death in epilepsy (SUDEP). The exact cause is unknown, but it may be due to changes in the breathing pattern or heart rate controlled by the brainstem. In the normal younger adult population, sudden unexpected death usually makes it into the news media, and happens approximately once for each 10,000 to 50,000 persons per year. In people with active epilepsy, the overall rate is approximately 1 per 1,000 per year.

Persons who have epilepsy severe enough to be treated with two or more AEDs, continue to have generalized tonic-clonic seizures, and who have mental retardation have 2 to 3 deaths per 1,000 per year are at highest risk for SUDEP. Persons who have well-controlled epilepsy with only a single AED have a much lower risk, which may not be much higher than the general population. SUDEP may happen during a seizure, but often it happens while a person is just sitting or sleeping. The emotional shock and feelings of guilt it generates can be difficult for the friends, relatives, and caregivers. These can be alleviated if the possibility of SUDEP is explained in advance to families of persons at high risk for this. It may never happen, but simply talking about this possibility—although much higher than in the general population—is still low, often decreases worry. Also, it is reassuring to know in advance that there are no known steps beyond good medical care that can be taken to prevent SUDEP.

APPENDIX 1

Answer to the question in Figure 1-7 in Chapter 1.

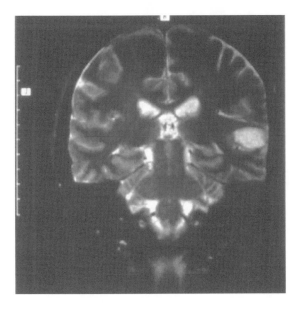

FIGURE A-1

The white roundish area on the left side is a tumor not detected by CT scan. The best way to interpret an MRI or CT scan is to compare one side with the other and look for differences.

Useful Sources of Information

General Information about Epilepsy and Its Treatment

Epilepsy Foundation (of America). This organization is similar to other disase-specific organizations such as the Multiple Scletosis society. It provides educational activities, research grants, and advocacy for persons with epilepsy.

www.epilesyfoundation.org

American Epilepsy Society. (AES). This is an organization for professionals whose principal activity is to treat persons with epilepsy.

www.aesnet.org

American Academy of Neurology (AAN). This is an organization for neurologists, many of who treat persons with epilepsy.

www.aan.com

CURE for Epilepsy. This is an organization started by parents of children with epilepsy and provides advocacy and research grants.

www.cueepilepsy.org

National Medical Library. This is the largest on-line resource for peer-reviewed scientific articles.

www.ncbi.nlm.nih/gov/entres

National Association of Epilepsy Centers. (NAEC). Most epilepsy treatment centers are members of this organization
www.naec-epilepsy.org

Americans with Disability Home Page
www.eeoc.gov/facts/fs-ada

Social Security Disability information for epilepsy
www.seniormag.com/legal/epilepsy

Glossary

Brain—The brain is an electrochemical organ that has billions or nerve cells (neurons) connected by axons and dendrites (biological wires) to other neurons or action cells such as muscle cells or glands.

Complex Partial Seizures—Complex partial seizures involve impairment, or loss of consciousness.

CT Scan—A very sophisticated X-ray in which a detector and X-ray source rotate around the patient. A computer then reconstructs the data into a picture on a screen or on film.

EEG—An instrument which detects very small electrical signals generated by the brain, which are detectable from the scalp.

Epilepsy—Epilepsy is a condition of the brain that leads to more than one seizure. It is the expression of abnormal brain activity during which the normal electrochemical processes are temporarily "short circuited."

Half-life—The time it takes for the blood level of a medicine to reach one-half of a previous level.

MRI—An MRI scan consists of a very strong magnetic field that is set up to hold the molecules in line while radio waves of certain frequencies are passed through the body. Detectors pick up the signals generated and convert them into computer displays or print them on film. It is more sensitive than a CT scan.

Seizure—A short, single event, lasting a few seconds to a few minutes, during which a person has uncontrollable strange or violent behavior.

Simple Partial Seizures—These are seizures in which consciousness is not altered.

Syndrome—The term is used to describe a collection of symptoms and findings from tests that identify a disease.

Tonic-clonic Seizures—These seizures are the most dramatic seizures which start out with the body being stiff (tonic) and then shaking (clonic). Also called convulsions and in the past known as "grand mal."

Index

NOTE: Boldface numbers indicate illustrations; t indicates a table.

RELATED PATIENT EPILEPSY TITLES
FROM DEMOS MEDICAL PUBLISHING

Keto Kid : Helping Your Child Succeed on the Ketogenic Diet
Deborah Snyder, DO
ISBN 13: 9781932603293, $16.95

The Ketogenic Diet: A Treatment for Children and
Others with Epilepsy, 4th Edition
John M. Freeman, MD, Eric Kossoff, MD,
Jennifer B. Freeman, and Millicent T. Kelly, RD, LD
ISBN 13: 9781932603187, $24.95

Epilepsy and Pregnancy
Stacey Chillemi and Blanca Vazquez, MD
ISBN 13: 9781932603156, $16.95

Epilepsy: 199 Answers: A Doctor Responds to
His Patients' Questions, 2nd Edition
Andrew N. Wilner, MD
ISBN 13: 9781888799705, $19.95

Growing Up with Epilepsy: A Practical Guide for Parents
Lynn Bennett Blackburn, PhD
ISBN 13: 9781888799743, $19.95

Living Well with Epilepsy, 2nd Edition
Robert J. Gumnit , MD
ISBN 13: 9781888799118, $19.95

Your Child and Epilepsy
Robert J. Gumnit, MD
ISBN 13: 9780939957767, $24.95

To order these or any other Demos titles call toll-free 1-800-532-8663, or visit us on the web at www.demosmedpub.com.

Demos Medical Publishing
386 Park Avenue South, Suite 301
New York, NY 10016